ALL GRAMMY'S TOP RECIPES
2nd Edition
Low Sugar, Low Fructose Alternatives
LARGE PRINT

Also by Kathleen Krauss Zucati

Bane, King by His Own Hand 2015
Larger Print

Destruction of the Talismen 2015
Larger Print

It's a Heckuva Life: 25 Years of Xmas 2015
Larger Print

All Grammy's Best Recipes 2015
LARGE PRINT

Adult Coloring Books:
Varmints & Critters & Pugs
While Away
Dark Visions, Bane, King
Dark Visions, Talismen
Dark Visions, Princesses

*Available on **a**mazon & **c**reate **s**pace*

All Grammy's Top Recipes
2nd Edition

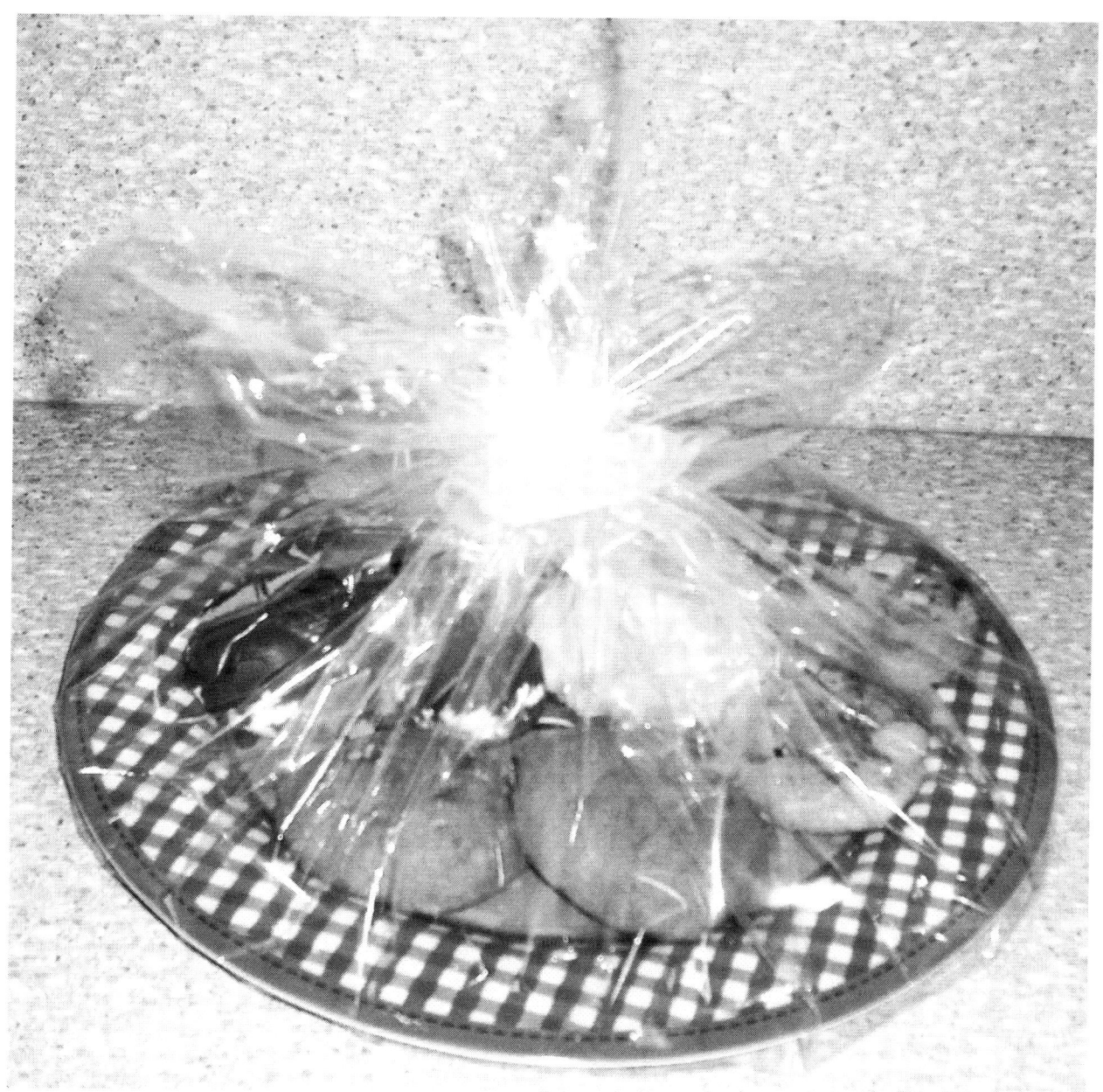

Low Sugar, Low Fructose Alternatives
Kathleen Krauss Zucati
With Paul E. Zucati
LARGE PRINT

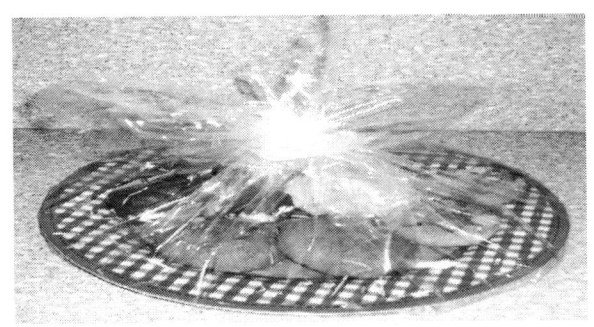

All Grammy's Top Recipes
2nd Edition
Low Sugar, Low Fructose Alternatives
LARGE PRINT

Copyright @ 2017 by Kathleen D. L. Zucati
with Paul E. Zucati
All rights reserved
Published in the United States of America
Second Edition ~ 2017
LIBRARY CATALOGING DATA
Zucati, Kathleen D. L. Krauss & Zucati, Paul E.
All Grammy's Top Recipes, *2nd Edition*
Low Sugar, Low Fructose Alternatives
Recipes, Cookbook, Fructose, Sugar, Glucose, Fiber, Health,
Carbohydrates, Carbs, Diabetes
Large Print
Non-fiction
The recipes in this book have been
tasted, tested, tweaked, updated and sometimes created
by Kathleen D. L. Zucati with Paul E. Zucati

.For brief review purposes and producing food, this book, its illustrations, and small portions thereof *may* be reproduced by any means *without* permission of the author.
You can contact the authors at:
thislldew@msn.com

Additional copies are available on **a**mazon and create space
This book is published on demand

*Dedicated to
Daniel Letinsky, M.D.
He knows...
He informs...
But he doesn't push.*

Glucose is fuel for the human body.
But humans have no known nutritional need
for fructose in any form.
	Dr. Robert Lustig
	<u>FAT CHANCE</u>

TABLE OF CONTENTS

About Sweeteners -- 9
Appetizers & Snacks -- 11
Beverages -- 16
Bird Food -- 18
Breads -- 19
Camping -- 25
Casseroles -- 28
Dog Food & Treats -- 31
Dog Food: Puppy Formula & Feeding -- 36
Eggs, Pancakes, & Breakfast -- 37
Fish -- 42
Fruit -- 44
Marinades -- 45
Meat -- 46
Pasta -- 52
Polenta -- 55
Potatoes -- 56
Poultry -- 59
Rice -- 63
Salads & Dressings -- 65
Sandwiches -- 70
Slow Cooker -- 73
Soups -- 75
Sweets: Desserts, Treats, & Snacks -- 80
Vegetables -- 88
Vegetables & Insulin -- 92

TABLE OF CONTENTS
Continued

Calculate Carb Grams per Serving -- 93
Camping Picnic Table Workout -- 94
Convert U.S. Measures to Metric & Convert -- 95
Counting Carbohydrates -- 96
Crafts (with food components) -- 97
Frying Oils & Fats, Smoke Points -- 99
Healthiest Foods 2016 -- 100
Picnic Possibilities -- 101
Poisonous to Dogs -- 102
Properly Balanced Meal -- 103
Recipe Versatility & Adaptation -- 104
Reducing Added Sugars & Fructose -- 105
Relative Dairy Fat Contents -- 106
Sixty-nine Names of Sugar -- 107
Suggested Reading -- 108
Summarized Fast Food Carb. Guidelines -- 109
Index -- 111

ABOUT SWEETENERS

All recipes for sweets in this book contain sugars.

These recipes *don't* include table sugar, brown sugar, or *fructose-containing* sugars. Free fructose may act as a slow toxin in humans.

The table on page 107, *Sixty-Nine Names of Sugar*, shows which sweeteners contain fructose and which do not.

But *all* sugars are carbohydrates and eating them can lead to weight gain and loss of diabetic blood sugar control.

Cattle farmers often feed corn syrup to their livestock for quicker weight gain and to add fatty marbling to make their meat tender and delicious.

It's uncertain whether it has the same effect in humans.

But in case it does, eat all sweets sparingly.

Karo syrup comes in several varieties:
1. **Light**: clear, 0g High Fructose Corn Syrup is stated on the front label.
2. **Lite**: has 33% fewer calories than Karo Light.
3. **Dark**
4. **High fructose corn syrup** (usually the largest bottles)

The *Sixty-Nine Names of Sugar* table on page 107 shows many names for sugars including *all-glucose* sugars. Any glucose sugars can subsitute for Karo Light, though you may need to adjust the recipes.

Type II Diabetes is easier to control when eliminating added sugars of all kinds. All recipes for Sweets contain "sugar," usually glucose.

To calculate calories, carbohydrate grams, etc., add recipe totals and divide by the amount eaten.

Foods like corn, flours, potatoes, etc. (starch) convert to glucose very rapidly, starting their conversion to sugar right inside your mouth.

Much more nutrition information can be found online.

APPETIZERS & SNACKS

Ham & Asparagus Rollups

Pickled asparagus spears
Thin ham slices
Whipped cream cheese

Dry ham slices and asparagus. Spread cream cheese on ham slices; roll each one around one asparagus spear. Use whole or slice and skewer pieces with toothpicks. ***Carb count: minimal***

Spicy Sweet Party Meatballs

Meatballs:
1 pound lean ground meat, pork, beef, or turkey
1 can water chestnuts, drained and diced
1 egg
1/3 cup whole-wheat flour (part can be flax seed)
1 teaspoon salt
1/2 teaspoon ground black pepper

Mix all ingredients, shape into 1" balls and set aside. Use a 1" round scoop, melon baller, etc. for uniform meatballs.

Sauce:
1 Tablespoon cooking oil such as real olive oil
1/4 cup chopped scallions
2/3 cup beef broth or water
1/2 cup Karo
1 teaspoon chili powder
1 Tablespoon cider vinegar
1 teaspoon ground ginger

Cook green onions in oil until tender. Blend in broth or water, Karo, chili powder, vinegar, and ginger. Add meatballs and bring to boil, reduce heat to medium. Adjust spices to taste.

Simmer 15 minutes, turning after 8 minutes.

Keep warm to serve with cocktail picks. Or chill and serve cold or freeze.

APPETIZERS & SNACKS

Dodo's Cheesy Bits

2 cups grated cheese
1/2 cup butter at room temperature
1 **scant** teaspoon ground black pepper (add **no** salt; cheese is already salty)
1 cup flour – may use 100% whole-wheat flour or other flour

    Mix cheese, butter, and pepper. Add flour. Will form a stiff dough. Shape into balls or sticks. Place on lightly oiled cookie sheet and flatten slightly.

    Bake 7 minutes at 400°F. Take out while still a bit underdone-looking. If you overcook, they'll melt and turn hard and dark at the edges. For chewy puffs, allow to cool five minutes and transfer to waxed paper or a cooling rack. For crispy, let cool in turned-off oven.

    Recipe will make about 30 round puffs and fills one cookie sheet.

    ~2 grams of carbs per "bit." 7-8 puffs equal one 15-gram serving

Chips

If you're going to eat chips,
The fewer ingredients and higher fiber, the better.

Juanita's brand corn chips with 0 grams added sugars, 3 grams fiber
Santita's ($2) chips with 0 grams added sugars, 2-3 grams fiber
"Bean" chips may be available. No sugar, 5 grams fiber per serving
Other brands and types of chips—read labels and find ones without sugar and with at least 3 grams of fiber. Chips have an average of 15 grams of carbs per ounce. Therefore, **about 6-7 whole chips make one serving.**

Salsaful Chip & Veg Dip

1 cup sour cream
1 cup no-sugar salsa, your choice of spice level (drain some liquid out)
Optional: small amount fresh minced onions, scallions, ground black pepper

    Mix well and serve.

    Cover and store up to several days in refrigerator.

APPETIZERS & SNACKS

Creamy/Dilly Dip

1 cup total of one or a combination of:
    Sour cream OR whipped cream cheese
1/2 cup cottage cheese
1 Tablespoon minced scallions or minced onions, your choice
1 Tablespoon chives (can be dried, fresh, or both)
1/4 teaspoon each garlic powder and onion powder
1/2 teaspoon black pepper
Up to 1 teaspoon salt
Optional: 1 Tablespoon prepared, no-sugar mustard
Optional for Dilly Dip: 1 Tablespoon dill weed

    Mix well. Serves as dip for chips, vegetables, chicken tenders, salad dressing, sandwich spread, etc. Keeps covered several days in refrigerator.
    Good with chips and crudités a variety of raw vegetables cut into in bite-size pieces or strips (next page).

Kimmy's Hamburger Dip

1 pound ground beef
2-3 cups homemade chili (no sugar) mashed a bit with potato masher
    OR 2 cans no-bean chili
½ small box original or spicy Velveeta cheese

    Fry the hamburger thoroughly and add chili.
Cut Velveeta into cubes and add gradually, melting as you go.
    Eat with thick or rippled potato or corn chips. Also good with crudités, a variety of raw vegetables cut into in bite-size pieces or strips.
    Easy to double.
    Very salty.
    Amount of sugar content depends on the chili you use.

APPETIZERS & SNACKS

Buttermilk Cheese Dip

2 cups sour cream (regular) OR cottage cheese, mashed with fork
1 cup buttermilk (add no salt; buttermilk is very salty)
4 – 5 ounces crumbled bleu, gorgonzola or other cheese, shredded
1/2 teaspoon ground black pepper
Optional: 1 Tablespoon chives (minced,)
Optional: 1 Tablespoon Worcestershire sauce
     Mix until smooth. Store, sealed in fridge for several days.
Good with crudités, chips, and on salads, baked potatoes, and sandwiches.

Crudités
(kroo-di-**tey**)

A variety of raw vegetables cut into in bite-size pieces or strips
Usually served with a dip or dips.

Asparagus (steamed)	Bell peppers
Broccoli	Carrots
Cauliflower	Celery
Cucumbers	Fennel
Green Beans (steamed)	Green Onions
Jicama	Mushrooms
Radishes	Snow Peas
Tomatoes	Olives, green/black

Add any other desired vegetables to this list.
Note: steamed vegetables should be well chilled before serving as a crudité.

APPETIZERS & SNACKS

Popcorn Two Ways
15 carbs per 3 cups popped

DIY Microwave Popcorn

Toss popcorn kernels in a plain brown paper bag, double fold the top of the bag. Pop as you would the processed kind.

You can also use a microwave-safe bowl with a plate on top to keep kernels contained as they pop.

(Or you can buy a hot-air popper.) **Fresh kernels work best.**

Pappa's Antique Stovetop Popcorn

In a Dutch oven or large skillet, heat about two tablespoons peanut or olive oil. Add 1/3 to ½ cup of fresh popcorn kernels.

Put a lid on top and heat on high, shaking and sliding the pan quickly back and forth as it pops. Keep sliding and shaking until the corn stops popping or slows considerably.

Take off heat.

Either: pour into a wire strainer to let unpopped kernels fall out (over sink or wastebasket) and put popped corn into a serving dish, OR simply remove popped corn carefully from cooking pot into serving container, being careful not to transfer unpopped kernels from the bottom.

Toss gently with real melted butter.

Salt lightly.

NOTES: Dogs may safely eat popped popcorn as a treat. Butter and salt should either be omitted or kept very light when offering to dogs.

No one should eat unpopped kernels (not dogs, not you).

Popcorn, while a reasonable treat, is not a meal—for the dogs or you.

Popcorn has about 15 grams carbohydrate per three cups popped. It also has about 5 grams of fiber per three cups popped, making it a "real" food according to Dr. Robert Lustig in <u>FAT CHANCE</u>.

BEVERAGES

Dodo's Antique Eggnog, Updated
2 cups cream AND 2 cups whole milk OR 4 cups half-and-half
Eggs (raw, 2-6, your call—wash eggs well before cracking open; you can also
    blanch by boiling for one minute before cracking, to kill germs.
3/4 to 1-1/2 cups Karo, to taste
1 teaspoon real vanilla or other flavoring
Nutmeg to dust

    Put cream and milk into blender. Add several eggs and sweetener (start with 3/4 cup and taste). Blend on low until lightly frothy. Put a half cup into a small glass, dust with nutmeg and there you go.

    If you're worried about salmonella from the raw eggs, wash first with dish detergent, blanch, or use homogenized eggs.

    This is a high calorie **dessert. Enjoy sparingly.**

Hot Cocoa, Aztec & Swiss
Aztec style—1 or more Tablespoons cocoa powder (can be non-caffeinated)
    Optional: 1/2 teaspoon chili powder (traditional for Aztec style)
    OR optional: 1/2 teaspoon cinnamon

    In a mug, mix cocoa and any spice to a paste with a little milk or cream. Add hot water, hot milk, or half & half to fill cup.

    Mix well. Whisking to a froth is traditional. ADD NO SUGAR—this drink is meant to be bitter, like coffee.

Swiss style—add NO spices, and add Karo to taste.

This is a food dessert, not to be confused with a thirst quencher.

    Swiss style has *15 grams of carbs per Tablespoon of Karo.*

Coffee & Tea
If you drink coffee or tea, drink them without sweeteners.

BEVERAGES

Juice & Carbonation
JUICE
Fruit juices have only *fructose* sugar, unless other sugars are *added*.
Juices should be taken lightly, including tomato and V8 juices.
Diabetics with low blood sugar should be treated with *milk*, not juice.
Whole milk (see below) is food, and helps hold blood sugars level.
If you lack vitamin C, eat a green pepper or an orange.

CARBONATED BEVERAGES
are implicated in some health issues.
Sugared soda carries a large carbohydrate load,
and sugar-free drinks contain artificial sweeteners—
but occasional indulgence in carbonated,
sugar-free drinks can be all right.

Milk
Milk is liquid food. As a rule, milk shouldn't be taken with added sweeteners.
Milk contains galactose / lactose (milk sugar) and has 15 carbs per cup; 19 for non-fat milk. FAT CHANCE suggests that you drink only whole milk, not skim.
(Note: too much milk can give dogs diarrhea.)

Water
Essential for health. The human body needs water every day.
Many bottled waters are not necessarily superior to local tap water.
Call your local water department to find out if you should filter
your tap water. If so, filter it. Filtered or not, keep a
container of tap water in the refrigerator for a quick, cold drink.

**Note: dogs need fresh water changed at least daily, in a clean bowl.
Birds also need fresh water changed often, especially in hot weather.**

BIRD FOOD

Hummingbird Nectar

1 cup very hot water
1/4 cup plain white granulated sugar
Optional: 1 -2 drops red food coloring (IS safe for hummingbirds now)

Mix sugar into hot water and stir until entirely dissolved. Add red food color if desired. Food color used today is not harmful to hummers. It's not *necessary* if you use a feeder with bright red components, but it's OK.

Let it cool before filling nectar feeders.

You can hang nectar feeders from your rain gutters near your windows by using a straightened coat hanger with hooks bent top and bottom.

In hot weather, change nectar at least every three days. It ferments fast.

Wash & rinse nectar feeder before refilling. It needn't be dried.

Hummers thrive on glucose/fructose. They also eat things like tiny bugs, grubs and tree sap. They make high-pitched sounds you can hear if you listen carefully. This nectar isn't harmful to them, and you may safely feed them year round. Only those species meant to stay in cold weather will remain all winter.

NEVER use low-cal or artificial sweeteners to make nectar!

Suet

Jays, grosbeaks, finches, and other birds will happily eat suet. So will squirrels, rats, raccoons, and other animals, such as your dogs.

Local butchers can provide beef fat trimmings. Cut them into small cubes. Melt in a frying pan or oven on low. If there are meat scraps in it, mince and leave them in. Most creatures enjoy extra protein. OR save drained meat fats.

Add your choice of sunflower and other seeds, small fruit, such as berries and sliced oranges, peanut butter, shelled, unsalted peanuts, unsalted walnut pieces, etc. Use baggies to package, shape into squares to fit in your suet feeder and freeze. Fill suet feeders as needed. More information online.

Some bird feeding guides suggest if you freeze & thaw suet several times, you can alter its melting point so it stays solid better in warm weather.

You can make a simple dog-barrier fence around the base of a suet pole or tree with a single 4 x 8 sheet of plastic lattice so dogs don't eat dropped suet.

Doggy NoNo! *Too much fat can give dogs pancreatitis, which can be fatal.*

BREADS

Holiday Bread Bowls

1 small round loaf of bread per person—use Whole Grain bread recipe and make each bread bowl 4 times as big as a single muffin.

Cut off top and save. Scoop out center of bread and save chunks. Fill with this mixture:

1/2 cup sour cream
1-1/2 cups grated cheese
1 -8-oz. pkg. cream cheese, softened
1/2 cup or more no-sugar salsa (your choice of spice level)

Wrap in two layers of foil. Bake up to an hour at 400 degrees; check after 40 minutes to see how it's doing.

Serve with chunks of bread and vegetables (crudités) cut into bite-size pieces, even meatballs. Use forks to dip. You can eat the whole thing.

High in fat and carbs—60 carbs per bread bowl.

Cornbread

1/2 cup cornmeal
1/2 rounded cup whole-wheat flour
2 teaspoons baking powder
3-4 Tablespoons Karo
1 Tablespoon real butter
1/2 teaspoon salt
1 egg
Up to 1/2 cup milk to make thick but not stiff batter
Add up to 1/2 cup rolled oats--optional

Mix well. Bake at 425°F for 23 minutes in loaf pan, or 18 minutes in cupcake papers. Makes about 12 muffins.

20 carbs per muffin or 1/12th loaf or sheet.

BREADS

Whole Grain Bounce
Rolls, Croutons, Bread Crumbs, Muffins & Flintstone Loaves
Too tender to slice. Fork-split muffins & small loaves.

1/4 cup vegetable oil, plus more for baking pan and oiling raw bread
2 cups hot water (bath temperature)
1/4 cup Karo to feed the yeast
3 envelopes or 2 Tablespoons any brand **rapid rise** yeast
1 cup old-fashioned rolled oats
1/2 cup flax seed or flax seed meal
4 cups whole-wheat flour
1 **scant** Tablespoon salt to taste

    Preheat oven to 350°F and generously oil or butter loaf pan, 8 x 8 baking pan or 2 cupcake pans for whole grain muffins.

    Place hot water, sweetener, and ¼ cup oil in a bowl. Mix well. Sprinkle yeast on top and let sit until the mixture begins to bubble, up to five minutes. If it doesn't bubble, it means yeast is too old or water temperature is too hot or too cold.

    Add oats, 1 cup of flour, and salt. Mix until just combined. Add the rest of the flour and mix until just combined.

    Oil your hands and form dough into balls. You can dip tops in sesame seeds. Put dough into pan (loaf or cupcake) or on cookie sheet in four balls for small round loaves. Cover with **plastic wrap** and let dough double, about 45 minutes in a warm place.

    Bake until skewer inserted comes out clean, about 45 min. for loaf, 30 min. for rolls. If you tap bread and it sounds hollow, it's done. Let cool in pan; *it will shrink*. Then tip onto a cooling rack. Freezes well.

    Croutons: cut baked muffins, etc., into ½" cubes. Toast in low oven until dry. This can take several hours. Put in airtight container like zip-lock baggies and freeze. Thaw before eating.

    Blueberry Breakfast Biscuits—add 1 cup small blueberries to mix.

    1 recipe makes 24 rolls, 15 carb grams each.

BREADS

Flat Bread

Breadsticks, Crackers, Croutons, Even Doggy Crisps
Makes 16 – 20 biscuits 450º F 10 – 12 minutes

4 cups whole-wheat flour
1/4 – 1/2 cup flaxseed
2 Tablespoons baking powder
1 teaspoon salt
1 stick real butter
1 cup shredded cheese (any kind)
Up to 1 cup milk (any kind, including buttermilk or almond milk)
Optional: sesame seeds, poppy seeds, kosher salt to top

In large bowl, combine flour, flaxseed meal, baking powder, and salt. Mix well with whisk or fork.

Cut butter into the dry mixture, using a cutting tool, two knives, or fork. It may look like pea-sized pieces of butter covered with flour.

Add the oats and cheese. Add milk and mix gently.

Knead the dough with your hands 6 – 8 times. Turn onto a lightly floured cutting board.

Biscuits: pat out flat and fairly thick with your hands until the dough is proper biscuit thickness, 1/2 – 3/4 inches. Cut into 2-, 3-, or 4-inch sizes. Coat with seeds or a sprinkling of large-crystal (kosher) salt.

Breadsticks & croutons: roll in poppy or sesame seeds.

Crackers: roll *very* thin and cut into cracker shapes.

Dog treats: roll thin and cut with a bone-shaped cutter.

Place shaped items on ungreased cookie sheet(s) and bake at 450°F 12 minutes for ¾" thick items, 8 minutes for crackers.

These burn easily.

Remove thick items as soon as lightly browned and cool on racks.

Allow thin crackers to completely cool in turned-off oven.

Can be frozen.

BREADS

Dodo's Celery & Onion Holiday Stuffing

8 cups dried bread cubes (white bread is best for this recipe)
1- 2 cups chopped celery
1 - 2 cups chopped onion
2 sticks butter
1/2 – 3/4 cup chicken broth (no sugar)
1 Tablespoon pre-mixed poultry seasoning
1 teaspoon black pepper
2+ teaspoons salt
2 eggs, whisked into a froth
Enough warm water to moisten

Chop the onions and celery and sauté slowly in some of the butter until they are *quite* tender. Add the rest of the butter and the water, the seasonings and spices and heat through.

Pour over dried breadcrumbs in a very large bowl, and mix a moment, then pour the whisked eggs over it all and mix well without crushing up the bread. Add water as needed to moisten all ingredients.

Stuff into a chicken or turkey and roast inside the bird.

If there's too much (and there probably will be) put the rest into a greased (oil or butter) metal bowl and cover well with foil.

Bake that for about the last 45 - 60 minutes of roasting time at 325°F, after untying the turkey legs.

Sugar/fructose levels depend on your choice of bread used. This tastes best made with dry white bread cubes, not whole-wheat. But if you bake the yeast bread recipe above, those crumbs work okay and you can eliminate fructose sugars.

NOTE: turkey flavored Stovetop Stuffing tastes almost identical to this dressing when baked inside a turkey, and is much easier, though less healthful.

BREADS

Bannock Bread

3 Cups flour
2 Tablespoons baking powder
Dash of salt
3 Tablespoons butter
2/3 Cup warm water (may vary)

Bannock bread is one of the most famous camping recipes in the world. Some eat it as dessert, some eat it for breakfast, some enjoy it as a snack.

The more you make it, the better you get.

Put all the ingredients except water into a bowl. Mix with your fingertips. You want the dough to feel breadcrumbs. Don't overmix.

Now slowly add some water and continue to mix with your fingers. You likely won't need more than 2/3 cup of water. Keep mixing with your fingers until dough holds together and is soft, slightly sticky, and bouncy but not wet.

To cook, fry in a hot skillet with a dab of butter until each side is crispy. Or wrap a bit of dough around a roasting stick and cook over an open fire. Keep turning it so it doesn't fall off the stick.

Not listed under CAMPING because it violates one of Grammy's camping guidelines: a good camping recipe should not be terribly messy.

Making this is quite messy. Work outside your camping rig or practice at home first. Have a bucket of water handy or a faucet to wash off sticky hands.

BREADS

A Few Store-Bought Whole Grain Breads

*Look for **3+ grams fiber per slice**, no HFCS, and low sugars. Note: yeast needs some kind of sugar to rise. If you bake your own bread, you can use Karo & eliminate all fructose. Many adaptable recipes are online.*

Arnold Natural 100% Whole Wheat
Dave's Killer Bread whole grain varieties, such as:
    Power Seed (6 grams fiber per slice with minor amount of fruit juice)
    Honey Wheat (5 grams fiber per slice)
    Blue Bread (4 grams fiber per slice)
    Good Seed (4 grams fiber per slice)
    21 Whole Grains (5 grams fiber per slice)
    Rockin' Rye (4 grams fiber per slice)
    White Bread Done Right (3 grams fiber per slice)
    100% Whole Wheat (3 grams fiber per slice)
    Sprouted Whole Wheat (3 grams fiber per slice)
    Dave's "Red" or "Green" breads (package colors), our faves
    And many more varieties including rolls and buns.
EarthGrains 100% Natural 7-Grain
EarthGrains 100% Natural Wheat Berry with Honey
EarthGrains 100% Natural Whole Wheat 100% Stone Ground
Food For Life: Ezekiel 4:9 Sesame   (in the frozen food section)
Nature's Own Organic Wholegrain All Natural 100% Whole Wheat
Pepperidge Farm 100% Natural, 100% Whole Wheat
Pepperidge Farm 100% Natural, 9 Grain
Pepperidge Farm 100% Natural, German Dark Wheat
Pepperidge Farm 100% Natural, Honey Flax
Sara Lee Hearty and Delicious 100% Multigrain
Sara Lee Hearty and Delicious 100% Wheat with Honey
Sara Lee Hearty and Delicious 100% Whole Wheat

          As a rule, bread is not a high fiber food,
Average of 15 grams carbs per slice

CAMPING
Grammy's Ideas for Great Camp Recipes:
- ❖ It has only a few ingredients
- ❖ It can be pre-prepped
- ❖ It needs only assembly and cooking at camp
- ❖ It's simple, innovative, and/or amusing
- ❖ It has few or no leftovers
- ❖ It is easily transported
- ❖ It can be cooked in a variety of ways
- ❖ It requires few pots or dishes or "appliances"
- ❖ It's easy to clean up

By these guidelines, "great" camping recipes are rare!
Also good cooked at home.

The simplest, most basic camp recipe is a can of cold baked beans; fancier: heat on a campfire. OR a steak cooked over an open flame.

Cowboy coffee is water, boiled in a frying pan over a fire, with a handful of coffee grounds thrown in and heated until it is nearly black.

Suit your camping recipes to your chosen methods of cooking: campfire with a park grill, your own grill, a park BBQ, hibachi, food on sticks, a gas cooktop inside your rig or set up on a picnic or other table, electric skillet, rice cooker, microwave, induction cooktop...there are so many choices!

New Breed of Dog
Microwave, campfire, or camp stove

4 – 8 hot dogs, chopped
1 can chili, your choice
3 tablespoons barbecue sauce, optional
Hot dog buns, gutted (save guts to add to chili or use as topping if desired)

Take all the ingredients, except the gutted hot dog buns, and mix in a bowl. Lay out each bun on its own sheet of tin foil. Fill the buns with the mixture and wrap the tin foil so the whole thing is sealed. Grill these over a flame for about 20 minutes. Put them deep in coals and cook them for 15 minutes. Timing depends on how hot you want them to be. Don't burn.

Can serve without buns

CAMPING

Hurry-Up Casserole
Microwave, campfire, or camp stove

1 package Ramen (type) noodles, well broken-up
1 ramen spice packet if desired (quite salty, but nice flavor)
1/2 cup water OR juice from a can of drained vegetables
1 can vegetables (drained)
1 can prepared beef w/gravy OR chicken or tuna (drained) (Ooptional: 1 teaspoon cornstarch)

Heat liquid to boiling in large microwavable dish and add ramen noodles and contents of spice packet.

Nuke another 3 minutes, then add meat and vegetables, and nuke another 3 minutes. **Makes two servings. Carbs: 26 grams/serving**

Double-Baked Potato Boat
Microwave, campfire, or camp stove

(Start by making a campfire or heating your grill.)
1 small, cold baked or raw potato per person (will need to be baked)
2 strips of cooked bacon per person
1/4 lb. sliced, cooked ham per person
Sharp cheddar cheese
Stick of butter

Cut each baked potato with 5 cross cuts. Do not cut all the way through. Into each cut, add butter, bacon, ham, & cheese.

Lay potato on a piece of doubled aluminum foil. Seal the potato in the foil.

Set in a hot area of your grill or fire and cook for about 20 minutes. Make sure you count the potatoes going in and coming out, as they tend to look a lot like darkened coals or charred bits of firewood.

Carbs—the potato: 1 small = 15+ carbs. 1 extra-large = 60+ carbs

CAMPING

Scrapple
(Leftovers Hash)
Microwave, campfire, or camp stove

For 2 servings:
1 cooked potato OR 1 cups cooked rice OR 1/2 of each
2 - 4 cups cooked meat
2 cups leftover vegetable or add canned or frozen veg of choice
Cooking oil
Butter
Salt & Pepper to taste
    Break up or cube meat and potato as necessary
Drain vegetable as necessary
    Heat oil in skillet over medium
Add dollop of butter
Add meat and potatoes or rice
Cook and chop up until bite-size pieces are crispy
Add vegetable and heat through
    Season to taste.
    Makes two good-sized servings for a complete meal
    Optional: fry a diced onion until tender in the oil, then add all other ingredients and fry until crispy

Carb amounts depend on potato, rice, and choice of veg

CASSEROLES

Bubble & Squeak

1/2 small head of cabbage, chopped
2 Polish, Kielbasa type sausage, in chunks (the squeak)
1 cup water
Optional: 4 medium potatoes, raw, sliced in bite size wheels

    Place all ingredients in a pot or frying pan. Layer chopped cabbage, potatoes, & sausage. Add 1 cup water, cover, and simmer until cabbage and potatoes are cooked—about 20 minutes.

    Servings: 4 big servings, 8 small
    Prep Time: 5 to 10 Minutes
    Cooking Time: 15 to 20 Minutes
    Carbs are almost entirely in the potatoes. They can be omitted

Harvest Casserole

Into large buttered casserole dish, layer, with cheese on top:
1 pound cooked ground meat, your choice
1 -2 onions, cleaned and well diced, sautéed until tender
4 - 6 stalks celery, diced, sautéed until tender
1 bell pepper, diced and sautéed until tender
4+ small potatoes, peeled and sliced
1+ zucchini, cubed or sliced
Red tomatoes, sliced
Yellow pear tomatoes, quartered
1 15-oz. can tomato sauce
6 Tablespoons butter or olive oil
1 teaspoon minced garlic
1 teaspoon ground black pepper
2 teaspoons kosher or sea salt
1/2 pound shredded cheese, your choice
Optional: 1 teaspoon Italian or other spices

    Cook at 375°F for about 90 minutes.
    Or layer all raw ingredients in crock pot and cook 4 - 6 hours on high.

CASSEROLES

Grandma's German Chili

1 onion, diced
1 – 2 pounds ground beef,
2 cans red beans, drained
2 cans black beans, drained
1 can lima beans, drained
1 can butter beans, drained, or 1 ½ cups frozen lima beans
1 -2 cans tomato sauce (no sugar)
1 – 2 cans diced tomatoes (no sugar)
1 teaspoon salt
1/2 teaspoon ground black pepper

    Sauté onion and ground beef in Dutch oven. Add drained beans, tomato sauce, diced tomatoes, salt, & pepper. Heat through.

    OR you can sauté the onion and beef and put them, the beans, tomatoes, and seasonings into a crock pot and cook on high for an hour, then low for 3-4 hours until bubbling.

*This chili can be used in **Kimmy's Hamburger Dip** and **New Breed of Dog** recipes...mash somewhat first. That way the chili portion has no added sugars.*

CASSEROLES

Southwest Casserole

In large, oven-safe pan or pot, in olive oil, sauté until tender:
1 yellow onion, chopped
2 scallions, chopped
1/2 bunch celery, diced or chopped
1 clove garlic, chopped or 1 teaspoon minced garlic
1 bell pepper, any color, cleaned & chopped
1 scrubbed, unpeeled chopped zucchini

After sautéing, add to onion mixture and cook through:
1+ cup diced chicken or 1 pound ground beef
Chopped or diced Roma tomatoes

Add to onions & meat mixture:
1+ cup cooked brown rice
1 can black beans
1 can corn, drained or 1 ½ cups frozen corn kernels
2 cans 14-ounce diced or stewed tomatoes with liquid (no sugar)
1/2 small package frozen lima beans
1 small can sliced olives, drained
1 can 14.5-oz. plain pumpkin OR 1 package frozen squash, thawed
2 teaspoons cumin
2 teaspoons kosher or sea salt
1 teaspoon ground black pepper
1 teaspoon taco seasoning

    Bake at 400°F about 45 minutes
.   Let stand 10 - 15 minutes and serve.

This can be made in a crockpot—simply put all thawed ingredients in, cook on high or low until onions are tender, several hours depending on your crockpot.

Carbs: beans, corn, pumpkin, rice

DOG FOOD & TREATS

Most Popular Human Foods 4 Dogs

Recipe for <u>Basic Dog Food</u> on next page. Raw fruits & vegetables may be diced or shredded after careful washing and trimming. No pits, rinds, seeds, etc.

- Albacore tuna, cooked
- Apples (no seeds) raw/cooked
- Apricots, no pits or trash
- Baby food
- Barley (no more than 5%)
- Beef
- Berries, fresh or frozen
- Bran cereal
- Bread, without raisins or nuts
- Broccoli (no more than 5%)
- Carrots, shredded raw/cooked,
- Cashews/nuts, **limited**
- Cauliflower, **limited**
- Celery
- Cheerios
- Cheese
- Cherries, flesh only, no pits
- Chicken, cooked, no bones or skin
- Chicken broth, no or low salt
- Chicken livers, gizzards, etc., minced, **limited**
- Cottage cheese
- Corn, cooked or popped
- Cream cheese, small amounts
- Croutons, plain
- Eggs, ***cooked only***
- Eggshell powder* (see below)
- Flax seed
- Fruit—flesh only, no seeds, stems, trash, etc.
- Green beans, cooked, drained
- Liver, diced or minced, **limited**
- Melons (no rind), limited
- Mint (helps with bad breath)
- Nectarines, no pits or trash
- Oatmeal, cooked in water
- Organ meats, giblets, tongue, heart, gizzards (no bones)
- Parsley
- Pasta, cooked
- Peaches no pits or trash
- Peanut butter, **limited**
- Peas, raw, frozen, or steamed
- Pineapple, fresh or frozen
- Popcorn, **popped only** no hulls
- Potatoes, **well-cooked only**
- Pumpkin, cooked or canned
- Rice, cooked, preferably brown
- Rice cakes
- Squash, cooked or frozen
- Sunflower seeds, unsalted
- Sweet potatoes
- Tomatoes, no green parts or trash
- Turkey, cooked, no bones or skin
- Yogurt, plain

DOG FOOD & TREATS
Lists of dog-safe "human" foods are online.

Be cautious of new foods. Offer in small amounts to start.
Cooked homemade food will keep in fridge up to three days; freeze the rest and thaw as needed. **(A list of Poison-to-Dogs foods is at the back.)**

Store-Bought Dog Food Feeding Guide

1. If packaged, must say, "Complete and balanced" on label.
2. Fat to protein ration should be no more than 50%.
3. Dogs need fiber and calcium as well as protein, fat, and carbohydrates.
4. No mystery meats like *Meat by-products* or *Meat Meal* etc.

Eggshell Powder

Save eggshells: wash well and let dry completely. Then grind with a coffee bean grinder or food processor. You can sift the powder through a sieve or strainer if desired. Birds love the larger pieces. Store in a closed container, and add to dogfood and treats before cooking.

Not only good for dogs and birds, but also good for you. It can be difficult to accept the eggshell crunch, so sift very well for people food. The powder can go into casseroles, baked goods, etc. 1 tsp - T in a people recipe is plenty.

Basic Dog Food
In a slow cooker (crock pot), combine:

3 – 5 pounds lean, raw minced or ground meat; beef, bison, chicken, etc.
Add 3 - 4 cups raw brown rice
6 - 8 cups water (twice the amount of raw rice)
1 Tablespoon or less kosher or sea salt & 2 - 3 Tablespoons eggshell powder
1/3 cup real olive oil
1/2 cup flax seed (usually available in bulk bins as well as packages)

Set slow cooker on high and cook until rice is tender, several hours.
OR steam the rice and fry meat separately.

In a very large mixing bowl, combine cooked meat and rice. Add other ingredients from safe list above. Occasionally include minced chicken gizzards for various nutrients. Let cool, mix and package in baggies by **SERVINGS: 1/2 - 2/3 cup for 20-lb. dogs**, then flatten the baggies for easy freezing.

To serve, thaw in refrigerator overnight.

DOG FOOD & TREATS

Doggy Cookies

2/3 cup no-sugar peanut butter
   OR liversausage / braunschweiger
   OR shredded cheese
1/3 cup olive oil
2 cups whole-wheat or other whole flour
1/2 teaspoon salt
1 cup raw rolled oats
1/3 cup flaxseed or flaxseed meal
2 Tbspns. eggshell powder for calcium
Up to 1 cup water to work
   Add water bit by bit

Mix well and shape into little bread sticks or flattened rounds.
Bake on cookie sheet at 450 F for 9 to 12 minutes.
Let cool in turned-off oven to dry.

Should be crisp, but not burned.

Check: *Safe Foods for Dogs* lists online &
Many dog treat recipes are online.
Poisonous to Dogs list at the back of this book and online.

DOG FOOD & TREATS

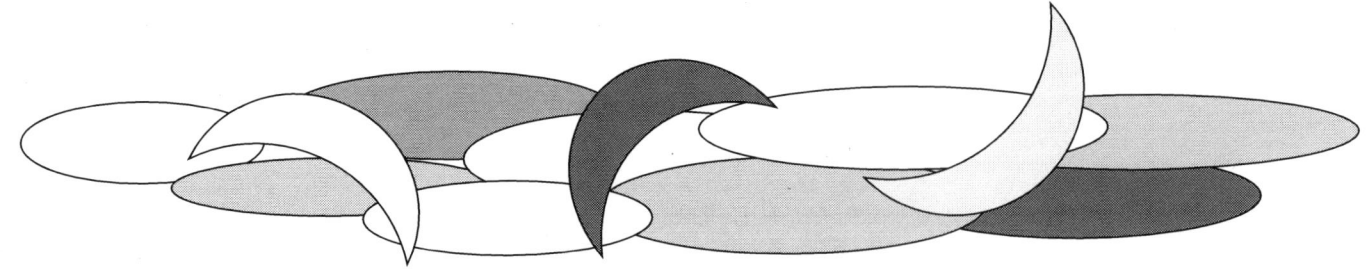

Sweet Yam Chews

2 medium-sized sweet potatoes or yams
   Preheat oven to 250°F.
Scrub potatoes, being careful to trim away any sprouts or green spots.
   Slice potatoes about ¼" thick.
 Arrange on lightly buttered or oiled baking sheet. Keep each slice separate.
   Bake for three hours or more until quite dry. These freeze well.

Pumpkin Treats

2-1/2 cups whole-wheat OR rice flour
1/2 cup pumpkin puree (not pie mix)
1/2 cup peanut butter
1/4 cup flaxseed or flaxseed meal
1 teaspoon cinnamon powder
1 teaspoon baking powder
1/2 cup water added as needed for proper texture to roll out

   Preheat oven to 350°F.
Mix all ingredients except water; add water sparingly to correct texture.
   Roll dough on lightly floured surface and cut into fun shapes.
Bake on cookie sheets about 20 minutes, and let cool in oven.
   (Yes, cinnamon is fine for dogs, but don't let them inhale the powder.)
   These freeze well.

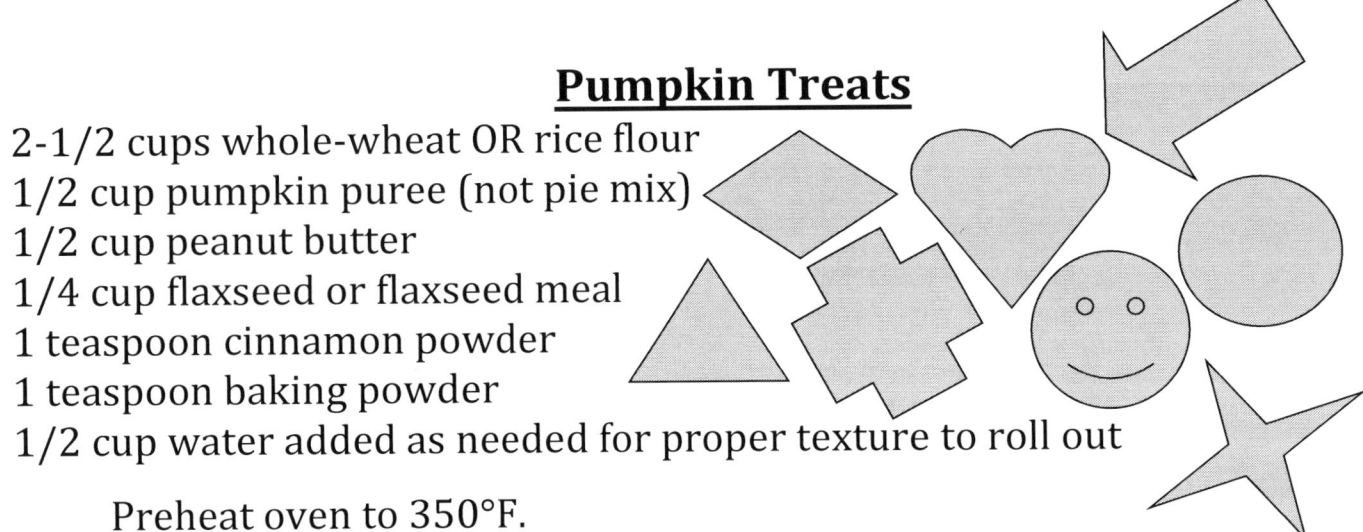

DOG FOOD & TREATS

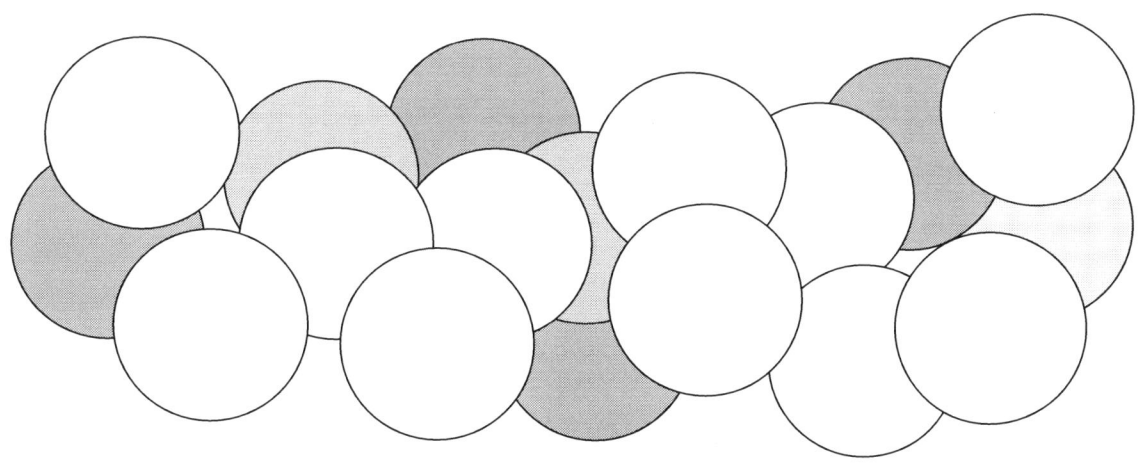

Hi-Pro Kibble Cookies
4 eggs
1 cup rolled oats, optional.
1 cup grated cheese
1 cup no-sugar peanut butter OR liversausage/braunschweiger
1 cup whole-wheat or other whole grain flour
1 cup scrubbed, finely shredded carrots, optional
1 Tablespoon eggshell powder for calcium

Mix well. Form into very thin sticks or little balls. Can use a rounded measuring spoon or small melon baller. If you want to roll and cut these, omit the shredded carrots and oatmeal.

Add more or less flour to make the texture right for forming or rolling & cutting.

Bake on ungreased cookie sheets at 450 F for 9 minutes.
Let "heat soak" by cooling in turned-off oven until very dry and cool.

As snacks or treats, give one or two a day for a 20-pound dog.
Very small versions can be used as training rewards.

Many dog treat recipes are online.
Check: **Safe Foods for Dogs** lists online
Poisonous to Dogs food list at back of this book and online.

DOG FOOD: PUPPY FORMULA
How do you make a decent puppy milk formula?

Supplemental or Replacement

10 ounces goat's milk (best) OR
1 large can evaporated milk plus 3 oz. cooled, boiled water
1 cup of plain full-fat yogurt
1 raw egg yolk (NO egg whites, ever)
1/2 teaspoon corn syrup ("Light" only, not "Lite" or HFCS)

    Mix the ingredients together with a wire whisk, place in a storage container and fill bottles to feed the puppies as needed. You can use regular baby bottle nipples to feed all but the very smallest (under 3 oz.) puppies. Don't allow milk to come out too fast; puppies can choke.

    Store in the refrigerator for up to 7 days. Warm the milk to body temperature before feeding puppies. Cold milk gives them colic. Discard any formula left in the bottle after each feeding; germs grow quickly in milk.

Puppy Feeding Schedule:

Newborns: feed every two hours around-the-clock for 3 days.
3 days old: feed every three hours: 5AM, 8AM, 11AM, 1PM, 4PM, 7PM, 10PM. Add a 1 AM feeding IF puppies wake and demand it.
5 days old: feed every 4 hours 6 AM, NOON, 4 PM, 10 PM. Add a 2 AM feed if puppies wake and demand it.
10 days old, feed 3 x daily, 5-6 AM, NOON, 6-7 PM
2 - 3 weeks old: Weaning onto solid foods *can* begin, and should definitely Begin by 4 weeks. It should take less than a week to complete.
From weaning on, feed 3 x daily through 4 months old.
At 4 6 months on, feed 2 x daily, breakfast and dinner.
    You can continue to feed 3x daily if you prefer.
    Divide total daily recommended amount by number of meals fed.

EGGS, PANCAKES, & BREAKFAST

Creamy Devilled Eggs

Boil half as many eggs as you wish to have devilled eggs.

Place cold eggs into pot of cold salted water and bring to a boil. Turn heat down slightly and slow boil or simmer for 20 minutes.

Remove from heat, rinse in cold water, and let cool.
Shell the eggs gently and rinse.

Cut eggs in half lengthwise.
Pop yolk into a small mixing bowl and use a fork to break up.

Add real mayo, sour cream, or soft cream cheese to moisten
Add kosher or sea salt & ground black pepper to taste. DO taste it.

Mix well and spoon yolks back into the egg halves (mound up). Use it all. Sprinkle with chopped chives, dust with paprika or ground black pepper, top with sliced olives, anchovies, almonds, hot dog slices, sausage balls, cubes of cheese, whatever you like, all optional. Perfectly fine to eat plain."

Spicy Devilled Eggs

4 hard-cooked eggs, shelled & sliced in half lengthwise
1/2 teaspoon salt
1/2 teaspoon dry mustard
Dash of cayenne (red) pepper and/or ground black pepper
1 teaspoon vinegar
1 teaspoon melted butter

Mash yolks with fork. Mix in all spices and butter. Fill the whites with yolk mixture. Garnish as desired.

Makes 4 servings, 2 halves each with 0 carbs.

EGGS, PANCAKES, & BREAKFAST

Quiche Eileen

1 flour piecrust, (Optional—if not used, butter a pie pan well for **zero carbs**)
5 – 6 whole eggs
1/4 bell pepper, cleaned and diced (optional)
1/2 cup mushrooms, diced (optional)
1 small zucchini, diced
3 green onions, diced
1/2 - 1 cup bacon or ham, diced and pre-cooked
1 cup shredded cheese
1 teaspoon kosher or sea salt
1/2 teaspoon ground black pepper

Sauté vegetables until tender. Beat eggs. Add everything else except cheese. Pour gently into poked, unbaked piecrust. Bake at 375°F for 45 – 50 minutes until center is set, then top with cheese and continue to bake five minutes until cheese is melted. Cool 30 minutes.

Optional: cooked celery, diced, cooked white onion, turkey, chicken, mozzarella, etc. Use whatever's available.

Pappa's Perfect Omelet

2 eggs per person, 3 if hungry
Butter for cooking and garnish

In a good pat of butter melted in a medium-hot skillet, fry whisked eggs until done and flip over. Grammy likes them a little browned.
Add fillings of choice and fold in half.
Serve hot with a bit of butter or the butter left in the pan, if any, on top.

Filled omelet—add diced, cooked ham, bacon, sausage, bell peppers, onions, shredded cheeses, mushrooms, tomatoes, chives, fine herbs, etc.

EGGS, PANCAKES, & BREAKFAST

Microwave Omelet

2 eggs per servings, 3 if really hungry or active
Fillers: cheese, bacon, sausage, ham, onions, peppers, chives, tomatoes, etc.
    Thinly spread butter inside a microwave-safe bowl.
Break eggs into the bowl and mix well with fork.
    Microwave on high for 1 minute.
Mix in desired fillers.
    Microwave on high for another minute.
Stir the eggs well.
    Add any cheese or other toppings now
Heat on high another minute if you want to melt cheese topping.
    Total time depends on your microwave's power.
Serve in cooking bowl or turn out onto a plate.

Dodo's Eggy Pancakes
(Crepes)

4 eggs, whisked
4 Tablespoons flour (can be 100% whole-wheat)
1 teaspoon non-aluminum baking powder
Enough milk to make a thin batter.
Coconut oil, heated until melted
    Mix ingredients well.
Fry quickly in a moderately hot pan, in coconut oil.
    Flip, fry quickly, and serve hot.

EGGS, PANCAKES, & BREAKFAST

Whole Grain Pancakes

2 heaping Tablespoons whole-wheat flour
2 rounded Tablespoons whole oats
1 heaping Tablespoon cornmeal and/or flaxseed
1 teaspoon non-aluminum baking powder
3 – 4 eggs
Enough milk to mix and pour
Coconut oil, heated until melted
    Mix well and fry in hot coconut oil. Makes 8 pancakes.

Pancake Toppings

1. Karo, warmed (can be tinted for fun)
2. **Drizzle** of sour cream or plain yogurt in equal parts with Karo
3. Fruit drizzle: small fresh or frozen fruit such as blueberries or raspberries sweetened with Karo
4. Whipped cream sweetened with Karo
5. Just pats of butter or melted butter – surprisingly good
6. Sliced raw fresh fruit or thawed frozen fruit

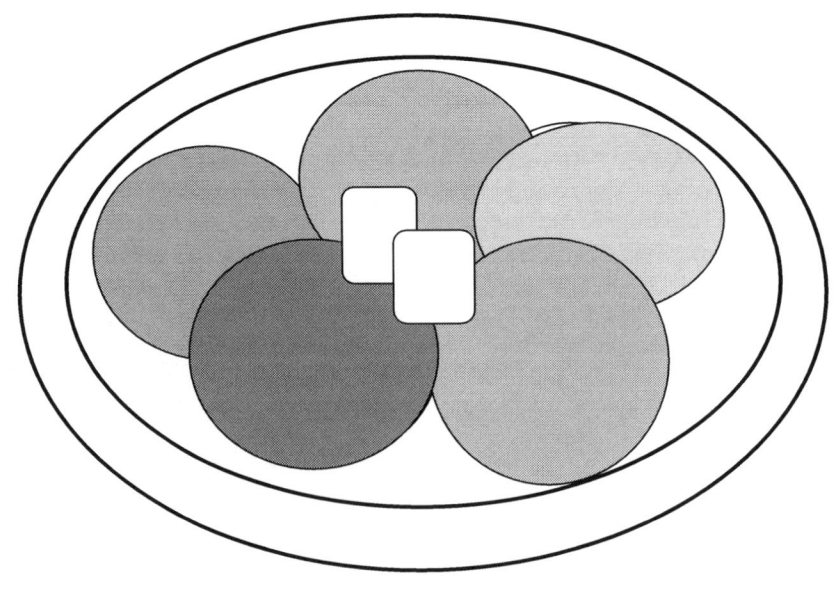

EGGS, PANCAKES, & BREAKFAST

Traditional Steel-Cut Oats

To make 1 serving:
1-1/2 cups water or milk
1/4 cup raw steel-cut oats
Prepare same as for 4 servings, below.

To make 4 servings:
4 cups water or milk
1 cup raw steel-cut oats

    Bring water or milk to a boil in a medium saucepan.
    Stir in oats, reduce heat to low.
    Simmer uncovered over low heat, stirring occasionally, for 25-30 minutes or until oats are of desired texture.

Crock Pot Directions

8 cups water OR 4 cups water plus 4 cups skim milk
1/2 - 3/4 teaspoon salt (optional)
2 cups raw, steel-cut oats

    Spray inside of 5-quart slow cooker with no-stick cooking spray.
    Combine water (or water/milk), oats and salt in the slow cooker. Cover and turn heat setting to LOW.
    Cook until oats are tender and porridge is creamy, 7-8 hours.
    Stir well. Cool slightly then serve immediately
    Can be set up the night before for a hot oatmeal breakfast ready as soon as you're ready to eat it in the morning.

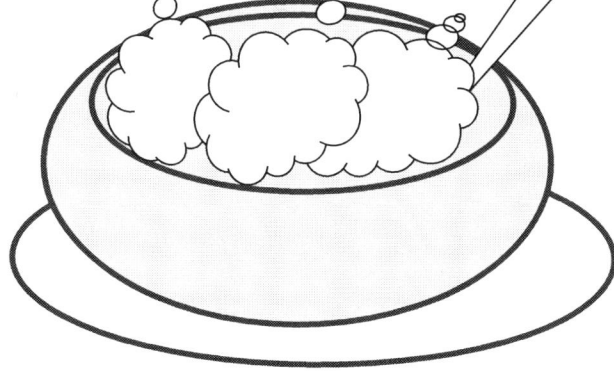

FISH

What kind are best to eat? Check "The Super Green List" and other sites online for recommendations of the most current, healthful, safest, & sustainable fish.

Unfishy Fried Fish

1 pound fish fillets
3 chopped scallions
1 Tablespoon soy sauce
Salt & Pepper
Lemon juice
Minced garlic

    Rub fish with lemon juice. Brown lightly in hot oil. Reduce heat & add onions & minced garlic. Fry five minutes.

    Mix soy sauce with 2 Tablespoons hot water, salt, & pepper, and a little more lemon juice. Pour over fish and serve.

Ahi Tuna Steaks

    Thaw tuna completely. Heat oil in medium skillet. Rinse tuna steaks but do not dry. Dredge in salt & pepper. Fry until bottom is white (2 minutes)

    Flip & fry until second side is white (2 minutes)

    Serve hot.

Broiled Salmon

1 fresh or frozen salmon
Salt &Pepper
Lemon juice
Olive oil & Coconut oil
Butter pats

    Rub broiler pan with coconut oil. Lay salmon skin down on pan. If frozen, let thaw 4 hours. Coat with lemon & oil. Dust with S & P. Set a few butter pats across top. Broil 5" from element 12 – 15 minutes. Peel from skin and serve hot.

FISH

Battered Fish Fillets

1 pound fish fillets, 1/2 pound per person, cleaned & completely boned
1 cup buttermilk pancake mix
1 cup flour, mixed w/1/2 tsp salt, 1/4 tsp pepper, 1 tsp baking powder
1/4 cup cooking oil

First step: heat the oil in a large skillet.

Clean and pat dry the fillets.

Dredge the fillets in the seasoned flour.

Mix the pancake mix and 3/4 cup water or beer, using a fork.

Dip the floured fish fillets into the batter.

Lay the coated fillets into the hot oil, only a couple at a time. Don't overcrowd.

Cook until the outside is golden brown.

Once the outside is done, the inside should be done as well.

Drain on paper towels.

Optional, sprinkle with dill, pepper, or lemon after frying.

Amount of sugar depends on amount in the pancake batter.

Breading is a carbohydrate. About 15 grams per serving of fish.

Baked Salmon

1 layer heavy-duty foil
1/4 cup olive oil
1/2 teaspoon crushed garlic
1/4 cup lemon juice
Dash soy sauce
Salt & pepper to taste

Mix; spread on salmon.

Wrap salmon & bake at 350°F. About 20 minutes per pound.

Flying Fish Sandwiches: See "Sandwiches"

FRUIT

Fried Apples

Wash but don't peel Granny Smith or similar baking apples, & dry. Slice sideways into rounds and core slices (or core whole apple first). Fry in hot oil 1 - 2 minutes per side until tender.

Replaces cranberry sauce, spiced apples in jars, etc., as a side, relish, or garnish. (Optional: dust with pumpkin pie spice or other spices.)

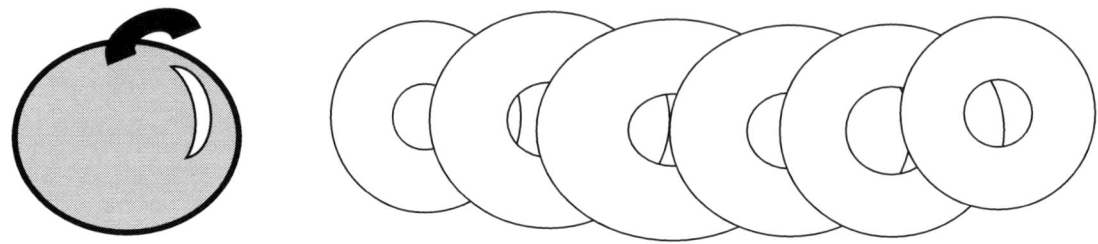

Whole, Plain Fruit

Fresh, raw fruit, possibly organic, washed but not peeled, has no added sugars, but contains fructose **with** enough fiber, nutrients, and micro-nutrients to cushion its absorption. Fruit *juice*, in contrast, has fructose **without** fiber, and is a hard "hit" on the human liver in much the same way that alcohol is a hard hit on the human liver. "Juicing" destroys the fiber by slicing it into such small pieces as to render it ineffective. This is true for tomato juice as well as other fruit juices. It's recommended that you, and especially young children, not consume fruit juices. (Dr. Robert Lustig, <u>FAT CHANCE</u>.)

Fruit contains carbohydrates and 100% fructose sugar.

Naturally-occurring fructose in fruit is part of a complex of nutrients and fiber that doesn't exhibit the same biological effects as free-fructose found in high fructose corn syrup (HFCS) and processed fruit juice.

Dr. Bruce Ames, Children's Hospital
Oakland Research Institute

**See the 69 Names of Sugar list on page 107
for help recognizing fructose-bearing sugars.**

MARINADES

Refrigerator Marinade

1/2 cup chopped green onions
1 Tablespoon cornstarch
1/2 cup non-sugar soy sauce
1/4 cup Karo
3 Tablespoons olive oil
2 Tablespoons sesame seeds
2 cloves garlic, minced
1 teaspoon ground black pepper
1/2 teaspoon ground ginger

Stir cornstarch, soy sauce, corn syrup, oil, sesame seeds, garlic, pepper, and ginger in a 13 x 9 inch baking dish until smooth. Add green onions, then add meat and marinate, covered, up to 24 hours. Turn several times while marinating. Drain and cook.

Cooked Marinade

1 Tablespoon cooking oil such as real olive oil
¼ cup chopped scallions
2/3 cup beef or chicken broth or water
1/2 cup Karo
1 teaspoon chili powder
1 Tablespoon cider vinegar
1 teaspoon ground ginger

Cook green onions in oil until tender; blend in broth or water, corn syrup, chili powder, vinegar, and ginger. Add meat and bring to boil, reduce heat to medium. Adjust spices to taste and cook until meat is done.

MEAT

Schnitzel

1 pound thin, boneless pork chops, thin boneless beef, or chicken breasts
1-1/4 cups whole wheat flour or fine breadcrumbs
2 teaspoons salt
1 teaspoon ground black pepper
Olive oil
2 beaten eggs

    Pound cutlets or chops as thin as possible. Mix salt & pepper into crumbs or flour.

    Dredge meat in seasoned flour, then in egg, then in crumbs or flour again. Fry quickly in hot oil. Serve hot.

Simple Enchiladas

1 package large 100% whole-corn or whole wheat tortillas (8 – 12, no sugar)
Shredded cheese, your choice
1-1/2 pounds ground meat
1 red pepper, diced
1 onion, diced
Olive oil
1 diced zucchini
4 + Diced Roma tomatoes
1 – 1-1/2 teaspoons salt
1/2 - 1 teaspoon black pepper

    Sauté onions, then vegetables, add meat and cook through.

    Roll scoops of filling in tortillas on a microwave-safe plate. Top with shredded cheese, heat through in microwave about 2 minutes.

    Filling can also be made in a slow cooker. Takes several hours.

    Filling can also be eaten without tortillas for **zero starchy carbs**.

MEAT

Modern Meatloaf

2 pounds ground beef
1-2 raw eggs
1/2 cup cottage cheese
1/2 cup Parmesan cheese
1/2 cup corn meal
1/2 cup raw rolled oats
3 diced scallions
3 Diced Roma tomatoes
1 shredded zucchini
1 small shredded raw carrot
1/4 cup flaxseed
1 teaspoon minced garlic
1 Tablespoon chives
1 Tablespoon parsley
1 Tablespoon salt & 1 teaspoon ground black pepper

    Press & flatten in loaf pan(s). Leave ½ - 1 inch of freeboard for grease.

    Bake at 350°F – 375°F for 75 minutes until crispy on edges and done clear through. Drain any grease before serving hot or cold.

    Optional: add chopped apple bits before baking, or shredded cheese either in the mix or on top.

    Leave out corn meal and oatmeal for **zero starchy carbs**.

Microwaved Bacon

    Place bacon on a microwave-safe rack or a plate lined with paper towels. Cook on 100% power (high) until done:

    Allow 1-1/2 to 2 minutes for 2 slices, 1-1/2 to 3-1/2 minutes for 4 slices, and 4 to 5 minutes for 6 slices.

MEAT

Pork Loin Surprise

1 - 2 pounds boneless pork loin
1/4 cup olive oil
1 Tablespoon salt
3 teaspoons black pepper
1 pound large-diced onions
1 pound cored and sliced Granny Smith apples

    Preheat oven to 375ºF.
    Toss loin with 2 Tablespoons oil. Roll in salt and pepper.
    Sear loin in large pan, two minutes a side.

Heat remaining oil; add onions first and later apples. Sauté until browned, five or more minutes. .Bake loin with apples and onions about forty minutes at 375ºF until onions are well done.

    Cover with lid or foil and let rest 10 minutes to set juices. Slice.
    Serve with onions and apples.

Sausage Suggestion

Find a store brand without nitrites, nitrates, or sugar.
OR:
1- 2 pound package of plain ground (organic) pork PLUS
1 large package Jimmy Dean, New York Style, or equivalent non-nitrite
    sausage, regular or spicy, with no added sugars if possible
1/4 cup flaxseed

    Mix thoroughly, divide into ½-cup patties, press flat in baggies, and freeze. Thaw and fry patties in a little hot oil. Watch closely; they burn easily.

MEAT

Mixed Meat Patties

1-2 pounds ground beef or bison
1-2 pounds ground plain pork
1-2 pounds ground turkey or chicken
1/4+ cup flaxseed or flaxseed meal
1 Tablespoons dried chives
1 Tablespoon onion powder
1 Tablespoon garlic powder
1-1/2 teaspoons salt
1 teaspoon ground black pepper
1 teaspoon celery salt OR paprika

    Mix well. Place by 2/3 – 3/4 cup in fold-over baggies and press well by hand until flat and square. OR—grill on hot coals.

    Freeze for up to 3-6 months. Can be thawed or fried from frozen.

Mixed Meatballs

Follow directions above.
Add:
1 egg
(Optional: 1/3 cup skim milk powder)
(Optional: 1 -2 Tablespoons flour; can be 100% whole grain)

    Cook by frying or nuking, and then freeze. To use, thaw, add to sauce recipe and heat through in pan or microwave-safe dish.

    If you don't plan to use them right away, freeze meatballs on a tray and then package frozen meatballs in baggies.

    Handy to have in freezer for quick snacks, meals, or hors d'oeuvres.

MEAT

Swedish Meatballs

1 pound ground beef
1 egg
1/2 cup fine dry bread crumbs, panko, etc.
1/3 cup finely minced onions (raw or fried)
1/3 cup skim milk powder
1/4 cup water
1 teaspoon salt
1/4 teaspoon pepper
1/4 teaspoon allspice
1/8 teaspoon cloves

    In a bowl, combine water and skim milk powder. Beat in egg and seasonings. Stir in breadcrumbs. Add onion and meat, mix thoroughly. Form into balls. Melt a small amount of fat in a frying pan. Add meatballs. Brown over medium heat; turn. Reduced heat and cook thoroughly. Remove from pan. Drain on paper towels. Keep warm and serve.

Serves 4.

    Top with pale gravy OR a simple sour cream sauce: Combine sour cream, milk, salt & pepper. Heat until just hot.

New Breed of Dog

2 hot dogs, chopped, per serving
2 scallions, chopped
4 ounces canned or leftover chili
1 - 3 Tablespoons barbecue sauce
1 hot dog bun, scooped out (reserve crumbs)

    Place all ingredients except hot dog bun (but including crumbs if you like) into either a small pot OR bowl and mix gently.

    Either heat in pot, scoop into both halves of hot dog bun, and serve, OR scoop into hot dog buns and heat in microwave.

    Optional: wrap in foil. Heat over campfire or among hot coals.

Omit hot dog buns for lower starchy carbs. 1/2 can prepared chili with no beans has about 20 carbs.

MEAT

Microwaved Ground Meat

1 pound ground meat crumbled into a 1-1/2-quart casserole dish.

Nuke, covered, on 100% power until no pink remains, stirring once or twice.

Allow 3 to 6 minutes for beef, pork, or poultry.

Drain on paper towels if desired.

Meat-Stuffed Acorn Squash

1 acorn squash
1 pound lean grass fed ground beef (or ground bison)
1 Tablespoon coconut oil, heated until melted
1 small onion, peeled and diced small
2 cloves garlic, peeled and diced very fine
3 Tablespoon balsamic or other vinegar
Onion or Garlic powder, or both
Salt & pepper
Cayenne pepper, etc., to taste

Slice acorn squash in half, scrape out seeds. Place squash face down on baking sheet. Bake at 375°F 40 – 50 minutes until soft. Take out, but leave the oven on.

Heat coconut oil in skillet. Add diced onion and garlic and cook until golden. Add ground beef and season. When it's nearly done, add vinegar. When the beef is finished, set aside and prep the baked squash.

Scoop the flesh out of the squash into a bowl. Keep rind shells intact.

Now dump in the ground beef mixture and mix. Re-fill the squash rind shells with the mixture.

Place re-filled rind shells back into the oven to heat for 5 – 10 minutes.

Serves two.

PASTA

Grammy's Best Lasagna

Fry and drain:
1 pound ground beef or bison
1 pound plain bulk sausage, no nitrites if you can find it
Now add and warm through:
2 14-oz. cans stewed tomatoes OR 1 28-oz. can crushed tomatoes
1 can regular diced tomatoes OR (optional: 1 box frozen spinach, thawed)
2 small cans tomato paste
1 Tablespoon Italian seasoning
2 Tablespoons chives/parsley
1 - 2 teaspoons minced garlic
1 – 2 teaspoons Italian seasoning, to taste
In a medium – large mixing bowl, combine:
2 pints small curd cottage cheese or ricotta cheese
1/2 teaspoon pepper
2 Tablespoons parsley/chives
1/2 - 1 cup parmesan cheese
1 teaspoon salt
1 pound shredded mozzarella cheese
6 – 7 eggs
One box of regular or whole-wheat lasagna noodles.
    OR 1 head raw cabbage, washed and separated. (no-carb option)

    Layer meat & cheese with uncooked lasagna noodles (or raw cabbage leaves). Bake at 350°F for 75 -90 minutes. *You don't need to boil the noodles or cabbage leaves first. They bake fine since other layers are fairly wet.*
    Top with more shredded mozzarella cheese and bake 10 more minutes. Allow to sit, covered, for 20 minutes before cutting to let it meld & set up.

PASTA

Green Cheese Rotini

Cook 2 cups dry, white or 100% whole grain rotini pasta according to package

Sauce:
1 fresh broccoli, diced OR 1 package thawed, frozen chopped spinach
1 teaspoon minced garlic
Olive oil
1 pound ground free-range chicken or ground meat.
1-1/2 cups milk
1 onion, diced
1 bunch scallions, diced
1 cup diced green bell pepper
1 thin-sliced zucchini, washed but not peeled
1 cup shredded mozzarella cheese
1 cup cottage cheese
1-1/2 teaspoons salt & 1 teaspoon black pepper
1 can sliced olives, drained
1 small can sliced mushrooms, or 4 – 5 fresh mushrooms, cleaned & sliced

Sauté bell pepper, onion, & scallions in oil until tender.
Add chicken and cook through. Add zucchini & any fresh mushrooms, and keep cooking until tender.
Add milk, cottage cheese, mozzarella cheese, broccoli or spinach, canned mushrooms and olives.
Simmer, stirring occasionally until sauce thickens, about 20 minutes.
Add cooked pasta, salt & pepper to taste.
Can sprinkle with parmesan cheese.

PASTA

The Family Spaghetti

Dry, white or whole grain pasta, cooked and drained

1 pound+ ground meat, beef, bison, chicken, pork, or turkey
1 diced white or yellow onion
½ bell pepper (any color)
1 large can tomato sauce (no sugar)
1 large can diced tomatoes (no sugar, with liquid)
2 teaspoons salt
1 teaspoon pepper
1 Tablespoon chives
1 Tablespoon parsley
(Optional) 1 rounded teaspoon Italian seasoning
1/2 cup grated parmesan / Romano cheese
1/2 cup mozzarella and/or cheddar cheese

Sauté onion and bell pepper in olive oil until tender. Add ground meat and cook through...draining is optional.

Add tomato sauce & seasonings and heat through. Simmer 30 - 60 minutes on low and add cheeses.

Serve over cooked noodles (technically, *spaghetti*, but you can use whatever style noodles you like).

All quantities of ingredients are approximate. Adjust as desired.

POLENTA

Cheesy Polenta

1-1/2 cups cooked cornmeal (1/12 cups cornmeal to 7 cups water)
    Follow package directions—or use a premade polenta roll.
1-1/2 cups sharp cheddar cheese, grated
1 stick butter
1 beaten egg
    Mix all ingredients together.
Divide in half and place in two, buttered loaf pans or casserole dishes
    Bake at 300° F for 45 minutes
This freezes well

What is Polenta?

Polenta is cooked corn meal.
Traditionally used as a pasta substitute in parts of
Northern Italy, especially areas that were Austrian before WWII.
It can be topped with most sauces including sweet dessert toppings.
Tomato-based sauces are one traditional style.
Polenta is also eaten plain, often buttered.
It can be eaten hot or cold.
It is traditionally turned out on a board after cooking in a pot
and cut with a taut string or cord held between both hands.

Note: cornmeal, like other starches, is a high-carbohydrate food.

POTATOES

Latkes
For each serving:

1/2 onion, cubed
1 large raw potato, cubed with skin
2 Tablespoon whole-wheat flour
2 Tablespoons chopped parsley or chives
2 eggs
5 Tablespoons dry milk powder
Salt & pepper to taste

    Blend in electric blender. Fry in hot oil like small pancakes.

Dodo's Antique Potato Salad

1 dozen small, clean, russet potatoes, boiled until fork-tender.
1 dozen eggs, boiled until hard (about 20 minutes)
Mayonnaise--enough to coat well.
2 – 3 Tablespoons of prepared mustard
2 diced pickles or 2 Tablespoons pickle relish
1 Tablespoon vinegar or pickle brine with dill seeds
Salt & pepper
1 teaspoon celery salt
Paprika

    Let potatoes and eggs cool.
Shell eggs. Reserve 1 egg to slice for garnish. Mix mayo & seasonings.
    Cut up potatoes and eggs into large bowl and add blended seasonings.
Mix gently. Top with round egg slices.
    Sprinkle with paprika. Chill and serve cold.

POTATOES

Cheddar & Bacon Potato Salad

8 med. potatoes scrubbed and boiled until tender, drained & cooled
10+ slices bacon, cooked crisp, drained, cooled and crumbled
8 green onions, diced
2 cups shredded sharp cheddar cheese
16 ounces sour cream or plain yogurt plus enough milk to make moist
1/2 teaspoon ground black pepper
1 teaspoons salt to taste
Optional: 2 teaspoons prepared mustard

     Cube boiled cooled potatoes into mixing bowl. Sprinkle with salt. Mix. In separate bowl, whisk sour cream, pepper, mayo, salt, and mustard.

     Add bacon, onion, cheese and potatoes. Mix gently & stir into dressing. Cover and refrigerate at least 3 hours before serving.

Twice-Baked Potatoes

2 well-scrubbed, small to medium potatoes, makes 4 servings:

     Bake or microwave until fork-done. Let cool until you can handle them easily or wrap and cool overnight in fridge.

     Cut in half lengthwise and carefully scoop flesh into small mixing bowl, setting empty skins aside.

Mix in well with potato flesh, using a fork:
1/4 to 1/2 cup shredded parmesan / Romano cheese, dried or fresh
1 Tablespoon chives, minced, dried or fresh
1 teaspoon salt
1/2 teaspoon ground black pepper
1/2 cup or more sour cream, cottage cheese, yogurt, even cream.

     Spoon mixture back into potato skins. Heat in microwave about 2 minutes.

     Can also reheat under broiler for a few minutes. Dust with paprika, black or red pepper, and serve hot.

POTATOES

Stuffed Potato Boats

1 medium well-scrubbed, baked potato per serving
Several strips of cooked bacon, crumbled
Sliced ham, diced and fried
Shredded cheese, any variety
Chives
Butter (whipped butter is nice)
Sour cream,
Broccoli flowerets, cooked

    Bake potatoes. When done, let set 5 minutes, then slice and spread open. Use fork to fluff interior. Add cooked broccoli, butter, cheese, bacon and ham bits, sour cream, chives, etc. Salt & pepper to taste. All toppings are optional. Add other toppings as desired. Each potato makes one meal.

Dodo's Potato Pancakes

For each serving:
2 medium raw potatoes, very finely shredded
Press liquid out between two plates. Then add:
1 egg
1/2 teaspoon baking powder
Salt & Pepper to taste

    Fry in hot oil and serve.

Microwaved Bakers

    Prick scrubbed, medium potatoes (6 to 8 ounces each) with a fork. Cook, uncovered, on 100% power until almost tender. Rearrange once.
    Allow 4 to 6 minutes for 1 potato and 6 to 9 minutes for 2 potatoes. Let potatoes stand for 5 minutes before serving.

POULTRY

Grandpa Gene's Chicken Cacciatore

3 – 3-1/2 pounds chicken pieces, with or without bones
Olive oil
4 ounces chopped mushrooms
1 medium onion, chopped
1 clove garlic, minced
1 Tablespoon minced chives
1 ½ Tablespoons vinegar
1 small can sliced olives
1 cup chicken broth
1 Tbspn. Italian seasoning
2 teaspoons kosher salt
1 teaspoon ground black pepper
1 large can tomato sauce
Optional: 1 Tablespoon fresh parsley, minced

    Rinse chicken. In a large skillet, fry chicken in oil to brown.
Remove chicken and sauté onion in drippings until tender.
    Add mushrooms and garlic. Stir in broth and spices.
Return chicken to pan.
    Add tomato sauce & heat just to boiling.
Reduce to low.
    Simmer up to an hour. Add olives & garnish with parsley.

Microwaved Chicken

    Arrange 12 ounces skinless boneless chicken in a baking dish, tucking under thin portions.
    Cover with clear plastic wrap, fold back one corner, leaving a 1-inch opening.
    Cook on 100% power (high) for 4 to 6 minutes or until thickest part of chicken is tender and no longer pink, rearranging pieces after 2 minutes.
    Makes enough for 2 cups cubed, cooked chicken.

POULTRY

Chicken Piccata

Preheat oven to 200 F, place a casserole dish in oven.

CHICKEN:
1/2 cup flour
4 boneless skinless chicken breast halves, pounded very flat
1 teaspoon salt
1/2 teaspoon black pepper
4 tablespoons vegetable oil (divided use)

Pour flour, salt, and pepper onto a plate and mix well. Coat both sides of the chicken. Shake off excess and set aside.

Heat 2 tablespoons oil in large, heavy frying pan over medium-high heat.

Sauté half the chicken without moving until lightly browned on first side, about 4 minutes, then turn and cook second side about 3 minutes. Transfer chicken to heated dish in oven.

Add the rest of the oil to the skillet and cook the rest of the chicken. Keep cooked chicken warm on a platter in low oven, about 250°F.

SAUCE:
1 teaspoon minced garlic
1 cup chicken broth
1 small lemon, halved lengthwise, then sliced
1/2 cup lemon juice (juice of one lemon) OR ½ cup apple cider vinegar
2 Tablespoons capers, drained
3 Tablespoons butter, softened
2 Tablespoons minced parsley or chives

In the same skillet, sauté garlic about 20 seconds, add broth and lemon slices. Increase heat to high. Scrape skillet bottom to loosen any browned bits. Simmer about 10 minutes. Add lemon juice and capers and simmer about five more minutes.

Remove pan from heat and stir in butter until it melts and sauce thickens. Blend in parsley or chives.

Serve sauce over hot chicken breasts.

Good with fettuccini or egg noodles on the side, and green salad.

POULTRY

Chicken Quesadillas

1 package tortillas of choice (large work best)
2 chicken breasts, cooked and sliced or diced in bite-size pieces
1 jar Tostitos salsa con queso OR 1 jar of cheese & 1 jar of salsa
1 can black beans, drained, rinsed, & mashed
1 cup shredded Mexican blend cheese (or choice)
Chili powder, ground black pepper
Sour cream

    Place one tortilla on a large plate. Spread 1 Tablespoon cheese sauce and salsa on the tortilla. Place 1/4 cup cooked chicken on that half of the tortilla.

    Spread 1/4 cup beans and about 1/4 cup cheese over the chicken. Dot sour cream on the chicken and beans, and dust with chili powder and ground black pepper to taste.

    Fold tortilla over and nuke 1 – 2 minutes. Cut into four wedge-shaped sections and serve; **can use guacamole, salsa, & sour cream for dipping**. *Makes four chicken quesadillas with 1/2 chicken breast and 1 tortilla each*

    Carb content: read package for grams in each tortilla. (Approx. 15 ea.)

Fried Chicken

Cut up chicken pieces, with or without bones or skin
1 cup flour
2 teaspoons salt & 1 teaspoon ground black pepper
1 teaspoon baking powder
Cooking oil such as olive or coconut oil, heated until melted

    Rinse chicken pieces and pat dry.

    In plastic bag, combine flour, salt, pepper, and baking powder. Shake chicken in the flour mixture until well coated. Refrigerate for 2 to 4 hours.

    Put and inch or so of cooking oil in a deep skillet. Heat to medium high, or about 370°.

    Place chicken in hot oil. When chicken pieces are browning well, lower heat to medium low. Continue cooking for 8 to 12 minutes on each side or until well-browned and juices run clear when pierced with a fork.

    Drain on paper towels and serve hot or cold.

POULTRY

Dodo's Antique 2-Step Chicken

1 cut up chicken
Salt & Pepper

    Fry chicken pieces in hot oil in **oven-safe** skillet until well- browned.

    Season, and place chicken in skillet into a preheated, 325°F oven and bake, uncovered, one to two hours or until falling off the bone. Good served with mashed potatoes & pan gravy.

Hawaiian Chicken Salad Mountain

1 large can cooked chicken, drained
3 ounces soft cream cheese
1 can drained pineapple tidbits, with juice
Toasted, slivered almonds
1 large box no-sugar Jell-O (your choice of flavor & brand)
1 cup water
Shredded lettuce or cabbage

    Boil water. Add Jell-O. Mix until dissolved. Add can of pineapple with juice and chill until set.

    Chop up Jell-O. Add broken-up chicken, well-mixed cream cheese, and almonds. Mix gently. You can add some of the shredded lettuce or cabbage to this, but chop first for shorter pieces.

    Serve with a scoop on a bed of shredded lettuce or cabbage.

RICE

Plain Rice Cooking Chart

Whole grain rice: Basmati, brown, Jasmine, long grain, short grain, etc. Some evidence suggests basmati rice has fewer carbs per ounce.

raw rice	water	salt	final quantity
½ cup	1 cup	1/4 tsp.	1 ½ cups cooked rice
1 cup	2 cups	½ tsp.	3 cups cooked rice
2 cups	4 cups	1 tsp.	6 cups cooked rice
3 cups	6 cups	2 tsp.	9 cups cooked rice
4 cups	8 cups	3 tsp.	12 cups cooked rice
5 cups	10 cups	4 tsp.	15 cups cooked rice

In sufficiently large pot for cooked amount desired, boil appropriate amount of water. Add raw rice, return to boiling, then cover and turn to simmer. Simmer for about 45 minutes until rice is tender.

Spanish Rice

1 pound ground meat
1 – 1-1/2 cup raw brown rice
2 - 3 cups water (twice the amount of raw rice used)
1 28-ounce can crushed tomatoes
1 tablespoon minced garlic
2 tablespoons olive oil
1 cup chopped onion
Optional: 1 cup diced celery
1 diced bell pepper, any color
2 teaspoons salt & 1 teaspoon ground black pepper
Optional: diced Roma tomatoes

Heat oil in Dutch oven. Sauté onion and bell pepper until tender. Add garlic & rice and sauté at least two minutes. Add meat and brown well. Add water, tomatoes, and seasonings and bring to boil.

Turn down and simmer, covered, 45 – 60 minutes until rice is tender.

Not as good in crockpot/slow cooker. Rice can easily become mushy.

RICE

Chop Suey

1 pound ground or diced meat
4 cups chopped or shredded cabbage
4 cups cooked rice
2 cups celery, diced
1 onion, diced
Cooking fat or oil
1-1/2 cups water
2 Tablespoons cornstarch
1 bouillon cube (chicken for chicken meat, beef for beef)
1/4 cup soy sauce

    Cook celery, onion, and meat in fat in large skillet until vegetables are tender and meat is cooked through.

    Blend cornstarch with a small amount of water, add the rest of the water and soy sauce. Add to cooked meat and cook over medium until thickened.

    Stir in cabbage. Cook 3+ minutes or until cabbage is tender but firm.

    Serve over cooked rice. 3/4 cup suey to 2/3 cup rice makes one serving.

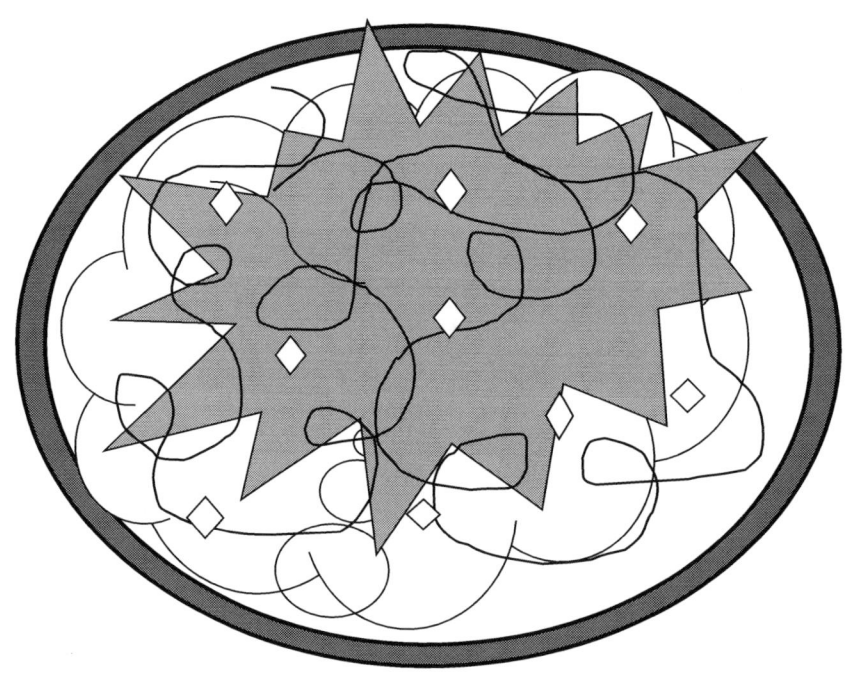

SALADS & DRESSINGS

Vinaigrette / Italian Dressing

1/3 cup white vinegar
2/3 cup olive oil
1 teaspoon salt
1/2 teaspoon black pepper
1 Tablespoon chives
1 teaspoon minced garlic
1/4 cup chopped scallions
Optional: for **Italian**, add 1 – 3 Tablespoons mixed Italian spices
    Blend in blender   Can be stored in refrigerator for a few days.

Creamy Ranch Dressing

1 cup of one OR a one-cup combination of:
    sour cream, buttermilk, cream, or mayonnaise (*not salad dressing*)
2 Tablespoons white vinegar
1 Tablespoon minced scallions
1 Tablespoon parsley or chives (can be dried)
1/2 teaspoon minced garlic
1/2 teaspoon black pepper
1 teaspoon salt (if NOT using buttermilk)
    Mustard Ranch: add 1 Tablespoon prepared, no-sugar mustard.
    Southwest Ranch: add up to 1 cup no-sugar salsa.
    Bleu Cheese: add crumbled bleu cheese bits
    Gorgonzola: add crumbled gorgonzola bits
    Bacon Ranch: add ½ - 1 cup crumbled cooked bacon.
    Mix, shake, or blend well. Serve over salad or as vegetable dip. Keeps for several days in refrigerator.

SALADS & DRESSINGS

Creamy Dressing

1 cup total of one or a combination of: Sour cream, whipped cream cheese, real mayonnaise
2 Tablespoons white vinegar
1 Tablespoon minced scallions or minced onions, your choice
1 Tablespoon parsley or chives (can be dried, fresh, or both)
1/2 teaspoon minced garlic or 1/4 tsp each garlic powder or onion powder
1/2 teaspoon black pepper & up to 1 teaspoon salt
Optional: 1 Tablespoon prepared, no-sugar mustard

Mix very well. Serve as dip for chips, vegetables, chicken tenders, salad dressing, sandwich spread, etc. Keeps covered several days in refrigerator.

Optional: 1 cup no-sugar salsa, lightly drained. Mix gently but well. Good with chips and crudités (next page), a variety of raw vegetables cut into in bite-size pieces or strips.

Buttermilk Cheese Dressing

2 cups sour cream (regular) OR 1 cup mayonnaise AND 1 cup sour cream
1 cup buttermilk
4 – 5 ounces crumbled bleu cheese, gorgonzola, or other, shredded cheese
2 Tablespoons white vinegar
1 Tablespoon minced parsley, fresh or dried
1 Tablespoon minced chives, fresh or dried
1/2 teaspoon ground black pepper

Mix until smooth. Store, sealed, up to two weeks. Good with crudités, chips, and on salads, baked potatoes, and sandwiches.

Salsaful Dressing

1 cup sour cream and/or real mayonnaise
1 cup no-sugar salsa, your choice of spice level
2 Tablespoons white vinegar
Optional: small amount fresh minced onions or scallions

Mix well and put into serving dish (es). Store unused portions in fridge.

SALADS & DRESSINGS

Pasta Salad Italiano

3 cups cooked tri-color rotini
2 cups broccoli flowerets
1 bottle (8 ounce) Italian dressing (this has some sugar, or make your own)
1 cup Parmesan cheese
1/2 cup chopped red pepper
1/2 cup sliced ripe olives
1/2 cup sliced green onions
    Toss together and refrigerate.

Crunchy Cabbage Salad

1/2 head cabbage, shredded
1 large carrot, shredded
4 green onions, chopped
1/3 cup real olive oil
1/4 cup white vinegar
1 teaspoon salt & 1 teaspoon black pepper to taste
3 Tablespoons Karo
Optional: sesame seeds, sunflower kernels, slivered almonds, peanuts
    Shred cabbage, rinse in warm water. Drain and pat dry. Chill in fridge. Mix all other ingredients and toss over chilled cabbage.
    Can top with crispy noodles, slivered almonds, or croutons if desired.

Greek Salad

Green pepper chunks
Tomato chunks
Onion chunks
Cucumber chunks
Olives, pitted
    Cover with ricotta or dry cottage cheese, & season with vinaigrette, Italian or Caesar dressing. Sugar content depends on dressing choice.

SALADS & DRESSINGS

Grammy's Caesar Salad

1 clove garlic, crushed & soaked in
1 cup salad oil at least 4 hours
1/2 head iceberg lettuce, broken
1/2 bunch curly endive, broken
1 cup croutons
3 – 4+ diced Roma tomatoes
2 beaten egg whites
1/2 cup parmesan cheese
1/4 cup lemon juice (small amount of fructose)
1 teaspoon Worcestershire sauce
Salt & Pepper to taste

After 4 hours, strain oil & discard clove. Pour oil over greens and tomatoes in bowl. Combine remaining ingredients and beat very well. Pour over salad and toss lightly. Garnish with croutons just before serving or at table.

May add sliced, boiled eggs, anchovies, or sliced olives.

Pappa's Basic Leafy Salad

In salad bowl:
Green leafy lettuce, 1 head, or red leafy lettuce, 1 head.
   Shred thick ends finely, chop or tear soft leaves into bite-size pieces.
Optional: 1/2 package fresh spinach. Cut off stems and chop or tear leaves into
   bite-size   pieces.
1 large or 2 small scrubbed but not peeled, shredded carrots
1/2 bundle rinsed and finely diced scallions
   Store in fridge in large lidded storage bowl with paper towel to keep crisp. .

SALADS & DRESSINGS

Andrea's Spinach Mandarin Salad, Party-size

8 ounces whole grain pasta, cooked according to package directions. Drain
4 cups fresh baby spinach
1/2 cup raisins
1/2 cup pine nuts (or peanut halves, or sunflower seeds)
1 4-ounce can mandarin oranges OR 2 - 3 sectioned mandarin oranges
1/4 cup cilantro, coarsely chopped

Sweet & Sour Dressing
1/4 cup olive oil
1/4 cup canola oil
1 teaspoon lemon zest (or fresh mandarin zest)
3-1/2 Tablespoons lemon juice (small amount of fructose)
2 Tbspns. honey (fructose/sucrose) OR 3 Tbspns. clear Karo (glucose)
2 Tablespoons peeled, grated ginger
1 clove garlic, minced
1 teaspoon Dijon mustard
Salt & Pepper.
 Garnish with chopped peanuts/slivered almonds/sliced boiled egg

Lovely Pea Salad

1/2 + bag frozen peas
1 cup diced fresh broccoli flowerets
6 scallions, chopped fine
2 – 3 lettuce leaves, shredded
1 carrot, finely shredded
Chopped chives – sprinkle
1 cup real mayonnaise OR sour cream
1 teaspoon salt & 1 teaspoon ground black pepper
Paprika and/or sliced boiled eggs to garnish
 Mix gently, garnish, and serve cold.
 Peas are a starchy vegetable and count as a carbohydrate.

SANDWICHES

Cold Flying Fish Sandwich

3 – 6 ounces of fish mixture per sandwich; sugar depends on bread choice.
1 small can of chicken chunks
1 small can of water-packed, chunk light tuna (or other canned fish)
1/2 cup real mayonnaise OR sour cream
1 teaspoon salt
1/2 teaspoon ground black pepper
Optional: 1 cup shredded lettuce or cabbage, or whole lettuce leaves
Optional: ½ cup shredded cheese, any kind
Optional: 1 squirt prepared, no-sugar mustard
Optional: Pickle relish, OR minced pickles—no more than 1/4 cup
Optional: no more than 1/4 cup no-sugar salsa

     Drain equal-sized cans of fish and chicken and put into medium bowl. Add pickles, salsa, squirt of mustard, and salt & pepper. Mix. Add shredded lettuce and shredded cheese. Add enough mayonnaise or sour cream for the texture and spreadability you prefer. Put dollops onto toasted, buttered whole grain bread and make two-sided or open-faced sandwiches.

Hot Flying Fish Melt

3-6 ounces fish mixture per sandwich; sugar depends on bread choice.
Equal sized small cans of chicken and tuna (or other fish), well-drained
1/2 + cup sour cream OR 1/2 cup real mayonnaise
1 Tablespoon chives
Salt & pepper
1/2 teaspoon each poppy and/or sesame seeds
1/2 cup shredded mozzarella cheese

     For melts, put slices of choice of cheese on top of open-faced sandwiches and broil or heat in microwave. Leave out shredded lettuce or put it on top as a garnish.

SANDWICHES

Basic Croque Monsieur
(croak mihsoor)

2 slices bread, your choice
1 – 2 slices ham, your choice
1 - 2 slices cheese, your choice
1 – 2 eggs, whisked (many online recipes offer variations, like cinnamon)
    Assemble sandwich using butter, etc. as desired
Dip into whisked egg, all sides, and fry in butter in medium-hot pan
    Many online recipes give variations including a liquid cheese option, various spices such as cinnamon, etc. But this is the basic recipe.
    Serve hot
Sugar level depends on bread and ham choices.

Basic Croque Madame
(croak madam)

2 slices bread, your choice
1 – 2 slices ham, your choice
1 -2 slices cheese, your choice
1 egg, fried in butter.
    Assemble sandwich using butter, etc. as desired. Fry on both sides, and lay fried egg on top. May be topped with cheese and broiled briefly.
    Many online recipes give variations including a liquid cheese option, various spices such as cinnamon, etc. But this is the basic recipe.
    Serve hot.
Sugar level depends on bread and ham choices.

SANDWICHES

Basic Welsh Rabbit (rarebit)
Per serving:
1 slice bread, possibly buttered, and topped with choice of cheese
    Microwave or broil until cheese is melted
    See online recipes for numerous variations, including spices, procedures, etc.; but this is basically *it.*
    Sugar level depends on choice of bread.

Basic PB&J
100% whole grain bread or use Whole Grain Yeast Bread rolls or muffins--
Adams or other non-sugar peanut butter brand, creamy or chunky
No-sugar jam or jelly, read the label ("Just Fruit" or "Simply Fruit," etc.)
Butter, just warm enough to spread easily
Optional: soft cream cheese
    Assemble and cut as you like.

Hot French Dip
1 large or several small French loaves (or your choice)
1/4 - `/1 pound of thin-sliced roast beef per serving
Butter
Beef bouillon cubes or beef broth in a can
Ground black pepper
Optional: onion, sliced thin & separated into rings
Optional: minced garlic
    Slice loaves horizontally and butter both sides.
Broil loaves about two minutes to warm and melt butter.
    Heat 1 cup water and 1 beef bouillon cube with 2 Tablespoons butter in a large skillet; simmer beef slices, onions, garlic, etc. about ten minutes.
Lift meat and onion slices with slotted spoon and arrange on broiled loaves.
    Slice diagonally.
Serve "au jus" (*with juice*) in small bowls for dipping sandwich.

SLOW COOKER

Roast & Stew

2 - 5 pound beef roast to fit in cooker
1 cup sliced celery
1 cup chopped onion
1 cup sliced carrots
1 Tablespoon vinegar
2 teaspoons salt & 1 ½ teaspoons ground black pepper
1/2 teaspoon minced garlic
Olive oil
1/3 cup flour whisked into 1 cup very hot water

 Drizzle oil in crock, place roast inside. Add everything else. Cook 4 - 5 hours high, 9–10 hours low.
 2nd or 3rd night, cube meat and veg to make stew. Adjust seasonings as desired. Add more water if necessary. **_Makes 8 servings_**

Bar-B-Que
Cook on Low 8 to 10 hours or High 5 hours

5 – 6 pounds boneless pork butt or shoulder, OR beef brisket
Choice of BBQ sauces:

A: Moderate
1-1/2 teaspoon salt AND 1 1/2 cups commercial BBQ sauce like Bullseye

B: HotHotHOT
1 - 2 14-oz. can diced tomatoes
1/2 – 1 cup white vinegar
2 – 4 Tablespoons Worcestershire sauce
2 – 4 Tablespoons Karo
1 – 2 heaping Tablespoons crushed red pepper flakes (to taste!)
1 - 2 Tablespoons salt
2 – 4 teaspoons black pepper (to taste!)

 Place meat in crock. Cover meat with (combined) other ingredients, cover crock and cook. When finished, shred or slice meat.

SLOW COOKER

Stroganoff
3-4 hours high, 6-7 hours low + 1 hour finish

2 - 3 pounds boneless meat sliced in strips, dredged in flour,
1 teaspoon paprika
1 teaspoon ground black pepper
2 teaspoons kosher or sea salt & 1 teaspoon ground black pepper
2 cups water
1 - 2 whole onions, well diced
1 teaspoon minced garlic
Fresh mushrooms, sliced
2 cups sour cream to finish—add only at the end

    Put all in crock-pot, cover and cook. To finish, add sour cream, stir well, and cover about 1 hour on low. Serve over cooked egg noodles. **_6-8 servings_**

Swiss Steak
3 - 4 hours high, 7 – 8 hours low

1-1/2 pounds beef round steak
1 teaspoon prepared mustard
1/2 cup flour
1 - 3 Tablespoons cooking oil
2 teaspoons kosher or sea salt & 1 teaspoon ground black pepper to taste
1 cup chopped onion
1-3/4 cups water
1/2 teaspoon minced garlic

    Cut meat into six pieces. Rub with flour and pound in flour with mallet. Brown meat in oil, add onions, S & P. Put into crock. Put water & garlic into pan and heat until boiling. Pour over meat, cover crock, and cook. Serve with mashed potatoes and at least one vegetable. **_Makes 6 servings_**.

NOTE: Harvest Casserole recipe also cooks well in a slow cooker.
HOT WEATHER: oven recipes can also be made in a crockpot.
    Carefully set up outside when it's too hot to roast or bake indoors.

SOUPS

Pappa Paul's Red Veg Soup

1 bunch celery, washed & well cut up
2 pounds carrots, scrubbed but not peeled and well cut up
1 onion, diced
1 bunch scallions cut up
1 teaspoon or more minced garlic
2 peppers, red or orange, cleaned and diced
2 cans diced tomatoes
2 cans wax beans, drained
2 cans tomato sauce (16-ounce)
1 cup whole grain pearl barley or brown rice
1 - 2 pounds meat, cooked, diced, ground, or shredded
Up to 4 bouillon cubes OR 4 teaspoons salt & 2 teaspoons black pepper
1 teaspoon each: chives, parsley, onion powder, celery salt, paprika
    Optional: canned water chestnuts, drained and diced
    Optional: red cabbage (1/4 – 1/2 head)
    Optional: zucchini, washed but not peeled, sliced or diced
    Chicken: boiled or steamed, pick as necessary & boil bones down, then strain and use bone water for stock. Dice or shred chicken meat.
    Beef: if using hamburger, fry thoroughly & drain before adding.
    In a very big pot, cover celery, onion, carrots and rice or barley with water and boil until tender. **Do not drain**. Add other ingredients and simmer until tender and flavors are blended, 40 – 60 minutes. <u>**Makes 12 Servings**</u>

Pappa Paul's Green Veg Soup
Differences from Red

No tomato sauce
Yellow or green peppers
Cabbage, if used, should be green, not red (1/4 – 1/2 head)
Canned beans should be green, not wax

SOUPS

Artesian Tomato Soup
1 can tomato sauce (no added sugar)
1 sauce can water (Optional: milk, half-&-half, buttermilk – or combo.)
Mix well and heat in microwave-safe bowls. Once you get used to this, you'll never want ordinary canned tomato soup again.
Add toppings like shredded cheese, ham bits, etc. ***Serves 2***

Alma's Pozole
Mexican Hominy Soup

1 large can hominy, drained
2 quarts water
3 large garlic cloves, crushed
3 bay leaves
1 onion – reserve 2 slices, the rest diced
1 Tablespoon chicken bouillon
2 chicken breasts
Oregano
Lime, cut in half
Shredded lettuce, 1/4 head
Sliced radish
1 - 2 teaspoons salt
1/2 - 1 teaspoon ground black pepper

Drain the hominy and rinse with warm water. Put into large pot and boil in two quarts of water with bay leaf until hominy is tender. Meanwhile, sauté the chicken with diced onion and garlic, etc. until onion is tender, then shred chicken and add all to hominy.

Add spices & bouillon to hominy. Serve with onion slices, lettuce, lime squeezes, etc., in separate bowls to add to your own bowl as desired to top off.

Optional: serve with Mexican crisp tostadas with sour cream and shredded Mexican cheese on top.

SOUPS

Clam Chowder
(Not Quite Max Ivar's Chowder)

2 - 3 (6-1/2 ounce) cans minced or chopped clams (reserve juice)
    OR 1/2 pound cooked, diced ham soaking in 1 - 2 cups water
1 diced white or yellow onion
3 – 4 diced celery stalks, *no leaves*
1 carrot, scrubbed but not peeled, diced small, about 1/4"
2 cups red potatoes, scrubbed but not peeled, diced about 1/2"
3/4 cup butter
1/4 cup flour (can be whole-wheat)
4 cups milk: half-&-half, whole or skim milk, buttermilk, or combo
2 teaspoons salt—none, if using buttermilk or only 1 teaspoon if using ham
1 teaspoon ground black pepper
Optional: Cooked, crumbled bacon on top
Optional: chives sprinkled on top – don't mix in—turns it green.

Directions

    Into a medium saucepan, drain the juice from the clams or water from the ham. Set clams or ham aside.
    Combine liquid with onions, celery, & carrot.
    Add enough water to barely cover and simmer, covered, over medium heat until almost tender, about 20 minutes, then add potatoes and simmer until all is tender. Set aside.
    In a pot, melt the butter.
    Add flour and stir into the butter.
    Slowly, whisk in half-&-half or milk.
    Cook and whisk until smooth and thick, about 5 minutes.
    If you want thinner chowder, add a little extra water, milk, or broth.
    Add the vegetables with liquid, clams or ham, salt and pepper.
    Stir gently and adjust the seasonings.
    Optional: sprinkle with crumbled bacon, minced chives, and/or pepper.

SOUPS

Fresh Broccoli Soup

5 quarts water in a large pot
2 Tablespoons kosher or sea salt
Ground black pepper
2 heads fresh broccoli
Optional: olive oil for garnish

    Wash & cut the florets and stems into pieces and put all the pieces into a pot with 5 quarts of boiling, salted water.

    Cover and cook for 3-1/2 - 4 minutes or until mostly tender.

    Use a slotted spoon; put all the broccoli pieces into a blender and fill halfway with the cooking water.

    Put the lid on and blend—careful, it's hot. Add more water to reach desired consistency.

    Taste; add salt if and ground black pepper as desired.

    To serve; pour gently into soup bowls; can add a drizzle of olive oil on top, can put shredded cheese in the bowl before adding soup, can garnish with croutons, crackers, chives, pureed red pepper, sour cream—whatever you like.

Fresh Carrot Soup

Follow broccoli soup recipe above, except:
Use up to 1 pound of carrots, scrubbed and cut up but not peeled.
Boil carrot pieces for 30-45 minutes until tender.

SOUPS

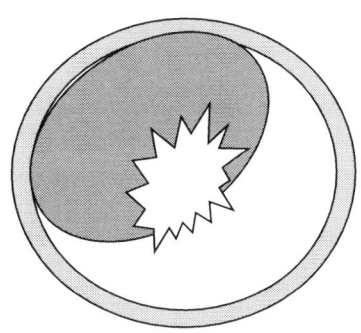

Cheryl's Yin Yang Soup

In microwave-safe pitchers, heat two different soups, such as tomato and split pea or clam chowder and red bean. Then pour them at the same time (one pitcher in each hand) into a soup bowl to form a two-soup pattern. Can give the bowl a quick half-twist to try for a yin-yang design. Can top with a dollop of sour cream, minced chives, etc.

Quantity of sugar depends on soups chosen.

(This is a style of presentation, not a recipe.)

SWEETS
DESSERTS, TREATS, & SNACKS
Low fructose does not mean low sugar.

Plain Cake

4 eggs
1-1/2 cups Karo
2 teaspoons baking powder
1/2+ cup whole wheat flour
1/2 cup oats
1 teaspoon vanilla
    OR 2 teaspoons cocoa powder
    OR other spice such as **Pumpkin Pie Spice** (below) for spice cake
    Nuke 11 minutes in 2 buttered microwavable cake pans.
Keeps well in fridge for several days.
1/16 cake = one serving

Mousse Cake

1 box cream or Neufchatel cheese, OR 1 cup sour cream
3 – 4 eggs
1 teaspoon non-aluminum baking powder
1/4 - 1/3 cup whole-wheat flour mixed in 1 heaping Tablespoon at a time
1 cup Karo
1 - 3 Tablespoons cocoa powder for milk-to-dark chocolate cake OR
    1 teaspoon plus real vanilla for vanilla or plain cake OR
    1 Tablespoon real lemon juice for lemon cake
    If batter is too wet, dust in more flour a little at a time.
    Mix very well. Do NOT blend or use cake mixer. Pour into 2 buttered glass microwavable cake pans leaving room for rising. Bake in microwave for 9 - 11 minutes. Check with toothpick for doneness.
    Let cool. *Keeps well in fridge.*
1/16 cake = one serving

SWEETS

DESSERTS, TREATS, & SNACKS
Low fructose does not mean low sugar.

Oatseed Cake

In a medium mixing bowl, alternately mix:
1 8-ounce box cream cheese OR 1 cup sour cream
1-1/2 teaspoons baking powder
In a smaller mixing bowl, mix well or beat lightly:
4 eggs
1 teaspoon real vanilla
Fold beaten egg mixture gently into flour mixture.
Gently add:
1/2 cup raw oatmeal (rolled and steel-cut oats)
1/3 cup flax seed
Optional:
1 – 4 teaspoons pumpkin pie spice
OR 1 – 4 teaspoons cocoa powder
OR other flavorings of your choice
    You can divide the mixture in two and add flavoring to one half.
    Pour into two, buttered, microwave-safe cake pans.
    Nuke each, separately, approximately 12 minutes.
    Advantages: lots of fiber, only glucose sugar, choice of a variety of flavorings.
    1/8 - 1/16 cake = one serving.

SWEETS

Cake Toppings
Drizzle
Mix equal parts Heavy cream, sour cream, or plain yogurt
& Karo and drizzle on top.
Optional: cocoa powder, spice, or flavors as desired.

Whipped Cream
Whip 1 cup cream to medium peaks.
Add flavorings, if any, to ½ cup Karo
Fold syrup into whipped cream.
Optional: flavorings
Mint
Cocoa powder
Pumpkin pie spice
Vanilla
Fresh sliced fruit/berries

See <u>Eggs & Pancakes</u> section for pancake toppings; also good on cakes.

Chocolate Flannel Moose

1 large prepared piecrust (or make without crust)

1-1/2 boxes of cream cheese, cubed & softened in medium bowl
2 Tablespoons cocoa powder
1-1/2 cups Karo
2 – 4 eggs
1 teaspoon real vanilla

    With mixer, mix corn syrup, cocoa powder, and cream cheese until smooth. Gradually add eggs and vanilla until smooth.

    Pour mixture into pie shells or two buttered pie tins without shells. Bake at 325°F for 45 - 70 minutes or until set. Cool on rack. Cover and chill at least two hours.

1/8 - 1/16 Moose = 1 serving

SWEETS

Grammy's 1967-2017 Apple Crisp
Alternative recipe for lower fructose

5 baking apples, washed, cored, & thin-sliced but **not** peeled
1-1/2 cups Karo (**Instead of** ½ cup white sugar AND ½ cup brown sugar)
1 cup whole-wheat flour (**Instead of** slightly less white flour)
1 teaspoon or more pumpkin pie spice (you can make your own; see below)
1/2 teaspoon salt
1 stick butter
Omitted: dredging apple slices in lemon juice after slicing

   Butter a square pan, dredge apples in flour, and lay in pan. Combine other ingredients well and pat over apples, pressing down. Bake 70 minutes at 350°F until brown on top and bubbling. Cool. Extremely sticky. Super with EZ no-fructose vanilla ice cream (below). (Original recipe was less sticky, was high in fructose bearing sugars and lower in fiber.)

1/16 crisp = 1 serving

Fresh Strawberries Luella

First, make a Vanilla Custard Flan Cake & let cool.
1 large no-sugar strawberry Jell-O with 2 cups boiling water, partially set.
Add 2 cups sliced fresh strawberries OR frozen sliced strawberries.
Fold in 1 pint whipped whipping cream sweetened with 1 cup Karo
   Chill 1 hour.
   Now fold in cubed Vanilla/custard/flan cake.
   Chill until set.

1 scoop (about 1/2 cup) = 1 serving

Note: fruit desserts contain fructose because of the fruit.
See carb counting chart for approximate carb gram.
For example, 1 small/medium apple = ~15 grams.

SWEETS
DESSERTS, TREATS, & SNACKS
Low fructose does not mean low sugar.

Very Berry Whip

1 tub plain yogurt OR sour cream (16 oz.)
1 cup heavy whipping cream, whipped to stiff peaks
1 cup Karo
Bag of frozen raspberries, thawed
2 cups frozen blueberries, thawed
Sliced strawberries

    Fold all together gently. Chill and keep cool in fridge.
        About 1/2 cup = 1 serving

Fresh Heavenly Hash

1 pint whipping cream whipped to stiff peaks
1 cup Karo, folded in gently to whipped cream
Add sections of mandarin oranges, peeled and cut in half or smaller
Add fresh cherries, pitted and halved
Add fresh pineapple tidbits
Add chopped nuts, any kind
Add berries, banana chunks, grapes, etc., all fresh
Can add cored but not peeled, chopped apple; it may turn brown.

    1 scoop (about 1/2 cup) = 1 serving.

SWEETS
DESSERTS, TREATS, & SNACKS
Low fructose does not mean low sugar.

Holiday Pumpkin Cheesecake Pie

2 plain pie shells, poked and baked at 325°F for 10-12 minutes
4 eggs, well whisked
1-1/3 cups Karo
1 cup plain canned pumpkin
1 rounded Tablespoon pumpkin pie spice (below)
1 8-ounce package of softened cream cheese, cubed

    Mix very well with mixer. Pour into plain pie shell(s) and bake at 325°F for 50 – 70 minutes. Don't burn. Cool on rack, then chill.

    May be topped with whipped cream, sweetened with corn syrup.

    1/16 pie = 1 serving

Pumpkin Pie Spice

1/3 cup ground cinnamon
1 Tablespoon ginger powder
1 Tablespoon nutmeg
1-1/2 teaspoons allspice

    Mix and store in an appropriate glass jar or plastic ware.

Autumn Ice Cream

Mix well:
1 cup plain canned or fresh, cooked pumpkin
1-1/2 cups Karo
1 - 3 teaspoons pumpkin pie spice to taste

Fold in gently:
1 pint heavy whipping cream, already whipped to stiff peaks

    Scoop into individual serving containers. Cover and freeze.

    About 1/2 cup = 1 serving & ~30 carbs

SWEETS

EZ Homemade Ice Cream

1 pint heavy whipping cream, whipped to stiff peaks
1 cup Karo, flavored as desired

Whip cream into stiff peaks. Gently fold in Karo. Add flavorings as desired. Cover and freeze in single-portion sized containers for 4 - 6 hours.
1 pint of cream makes 12 servings of 30 carbohydrate grams each.
About 1/2 cup = 1 serving & ~30 carbs

Flavors 4 Ice Cream or Toppings

Add to corn syrup.

Almond: 1 - 2 teaspoons almond flavor + slivered almonds.
Berry: sliced larger berries, or whole, small berries. About 1 cup.
Chocolate: 1 – 3 Tbspns. cocoa powder. Garnish w/ baking chocolate curls
Chocolate mint: cocoa powder plus 1 - 2 teaspoons of mint flavor.
Coconut: unthinkable. But if you do think of it, fold in last.
Hot dog: truly unthinkable.
Mega-watt chocolate strawberry berry mint almond: all that
Mint: 1 - 2 teaspoons peppermint, spearmint, etc.
Peanut butter: add 1/2 cup peanut butter to Karo before folding in.
Strawberry almond
Very Berry: mix of several kinds of berries, bigger ones sliced.
Very Vanilla: add 1 or more teaspoons real vanilla flavoring. Can tint.

Relative Cost 4 Ice Cream:

Brand	Price (1.5 quarts)
Store brand	$3.58 (20% less cost)
Homemade	$4.49
Breyers	$6.17 (37% more cost)
Ben & Jerry's	$14.85 (231% more cost)
Häagen-Dazs	$17.11 (281% more cost)

SWEETS

Cheesecake, Three Ways

ONE: Custard Style cheesecake
1-1/2 8-ounce packages of softened cream cheese
2 – 3 eggs
1-1/3 cups Karo
1 Tablespoon real vanilla
1/4 cup heavy cream

    In bowl on high, mix eggs, Karo, vanilla and cream. Add cubed cream cheese slowly until mixture is smooth.

    Fill two buttered pie tins or two pie shells and bake 45 minutes at 325°F until just firm. Cool on rack and chill.   1/16 total = 1 serving

TWO:* C*ake Style cheesecake
    After mixing as above, add
1/2 cup cornstarch OR ½ cup whole-wheat flour
1 teaspoon non-aluminum baking powder
1/2 cup finely shredded cheddar cheese

    Mix very well on high and bake in two buttered pie tins or pie shells 45 minutes at 325°F.   1/16 total = 1 serving

THREE: Both Worlds (custard style ***and*** cake style)
    After mixing custard-style #1 above, pour half plus 2 Tablespoons into a buttered pie tin or pie shell. Reserve. Leave the rest in mixing bowl and add
    1/4 cup cornstarch OR ¼ cup whole-wheat flour
    1 teaspoon non-aluminum baking powder
    1/2 cup finely shredded cheddar cheese

    Mix very well on high. Pour into a second buttered pan or pie shell and bake both cakes 45 minutes at 325°F.   1/16 total = 1 serving

Cheesecake Toppings

Whip heavy cream into stiff peaks and sweeten with Karo.
You can top with fresh berries, dust with nutmeg, etc.
Drizzle sparingly with plain Karo or equal parts Karo + sour cream

VEGETABLES

Roasted Brussels Sprouts

Preheat oven to 425°F

Rinse well an amount of Brussels sprouts to eat in one meal.
Slice Brussels sprouts thinly.
Toss in bowl with
2 Tablespoons olive oil
Salt **lightly**, no more than 1 teaspoon
Sprinkle with ground black pepper
  Lightly oil a cookie sheet and spread sprouts on top.
  Bake until brown, about 20 minutes. Cool five minutes and serve.
Be careful not to burn. Best eaten freshly hot.

Cheese-Stuffed Mushrooms

6 very large fresh mushrooms well cleaned
  Pull out stems & chop.
  Stuff hollowed mushrooms with mixture of:
Shredded or grated cheeses
Parmesan cheese
Cottage cheese
½ teaspoon chopped chives
1 teaspoon chopped green onion
Chopped mushroom stems
Bit of minced or crushed garlic
Salt & black pepper
Sprinkle top with paprika
  Bake at 400°F on oiled cookie sheet for 25 minutes. Best eaten hot.

Easy-Peasy Coleslaw

Shred fresh cabbage – red or green
Shred one well-scrubbed carrot
Top with commercial coleslaw dressing mixed with at least 2 Tablespoons of white vinegar
  Dust with ground black pepper, optional

VEGETABLES

Cheesy Beans

Canned wax or green beans, drained (may use fresh steamed beans)
Butter (~1 Tablespoon)
Shredded cheese (enough to complement the amount of beans used)
Slivered almonds (sprinkle over the top before nuking)
Ground black pepper (a nice sprinkling)

    Layer ingredients in order in a microwave safe dish and heat 1 minute or more until cheese is lightly melted. May stir or not before serving.

Multi-Bean Salad
(3-Bean Salad)

In a larger, shallow bowl, dish, or pan, combine:
3 cans green beans, drained
1 can wax beans, drained
1 small can sliced olives
1 can water chestnuts, drained and julienned
Optional: 1 can black, garbanzo, OR baby lima beans, etc., drained & rinsed

    In a small bowl, whisk well and pour over vegetables:
1/2 cup real olive oil
1/2 cup Karo
1/2 cup white vinegar
1 Tablespoon chives
1 teaspoon salt
1 teaspoon garlic powder
1 teaspoon onion powder
1/2 teaspoon ground black pepper to taste

    Push vegetables gently into liquid and cover. Refrigerate/marinate at least two hours, stirring occasionally. Even better if left overnight.

    Keeps well in fridge for several days.

VEGETABLES

Cooking Chart (time in minutes)

VEGETABLE	STEAM	NUKE	BLANCH	BOIL	OTHER
Artichoke, hearts	10—15	6—7	8—12	10—15	Stir-fry 10
Artichoke, whole	30—60	4—5	N/A	25—40	N/A
Asparagus	8 – 10	4—6	2—3	5—12	Stir-fry 5
Beets	40—60	14—18	N/A	30—60	Bake 60/350°F
Broccoli florets	5—6	4—5	2—3	4—5	Stir-fry 3—4
Brussels sprouts	6—12	7—8	4—5	5—10	Halve, stir-fry 3--4
Cabbage, shredded	5—8	8—10	N/A	5—10	Stir-fry 3—4
Cabbage, wedges	6—9	10—12	N/A	10—15	Blanch, stuff, bake
Carrots, sliced	4—5	4—7	3—4	5—10	Stir-fry 3--4
Carrots, whole	10—15	8—10	4—5	15—20	Bake 30-40/350°F
Cauliflower, florets	6—10	3—4	3—4	5—8	Sir-fry 3—4
Cauliflower, whole	15—20	6—7	4—5	10—15	Blanch, then 20/350°F
Corn, on cob	6—10	3—4	3—4	4—7	Soak 10, bake 375°F
Corn, cut	4—6	2	2 ½--4	3—4	Stir-fry 3—4
Eggplant, diced	5—6	5—6	3—4	5—10	Bake 10—15 at 425°F
Eggplant, whole	15—30	7—10	10—15	10—15	Bake 30 at 400°F
Green beans	5—15	6—12	4—5	10-20	Stir-fry 3—4
Greens: collard, mustard, turnip	NR	18—20	8—15	30—60	Stir-fry mustard greens 4—6
Kale	4—6	8—10	4—5	5—8	Stir-fry 2--3
Kohlrabi	35	8—12	N/A	15-30	Bake 55 at 350°F

VEGETABLE	STEAM	NUKE	BLANCH	BOIL	OTHER
Mushrooms	4—5	3—4	N/A	3—4 in broth	Stir-fry, broil 4—5
Onions, pearl	15—20	5—7	2—3	10—20	Braise in broth 15—20
Onions, whole	20—25	6—10	N/A	20—30	Bake 60/400°F
Parsnips	8—10	4—6	3—4	5—10	Bake 30 at 325°F
Peas	3—5	5—7	1—2	8—12	Stir-fry 2—3
Peppers, bell	2—4	2—4	2—3	4—5	Stir-fry 2—3
Potatoes, cut	10—12	8—10	N/A	15—20	Bake 25—30 400°F
Potatoes, whole	*12—30*	6—8	N/A	20—30	Bake 40—60 at 400°F
Spinach	5—6	3—4	2—3	2—5	Stir-fry 3
Squash, halves	15—40	6—10	N/A	5—10	Bake 40—60 375°F
Squash, sliced	5—10	3—6	2---3	5—10	N/A
Squash, whole	NR	5—6	N/A	20—30	Bake 40—90 at 350°F
Tomatoes	2—3	3—4	1—2	N/A	Bake halves 8—15 at 400°F
Turnips, cubed	12—15	6—8	2—3	5—8	Stir-fry 2—3
Turnips, whole	20—25	9—12	N/A	15—20	Bake 30—45 at 350°F
Zucchini	5—10	3—6	2—3	5—10	Broil halves 5

VEGETABLES & INSULIN

Non-Starch: Need No Insulin
Asparagus
Broccoli
Brussels sprouts
Cabbage
Carrots
Cauliflower
Mushrooms
Onions
String (green) beans
Tomatoes
Zucchini

Recipes:
Cheesy String Beans
Toasted Brussels Sprouts

Starchy, Insulin Required
Broad beans (red, black, etc.)
Corn, cornmeal, corn chips, etc.
Peas including split peas
Potatoes, potato chips, etc.
Breaded Vegetables

CALCULATE CARBOHYDRATE GRAMS PER SERVING

For any carbohydrate food or recipe (see Counting Carbohydrates list and check product labels), you can calculate approximately how many carbs each serving contains. Here's how:

Using product labels or information from CalorieKing.com or other food values information site online, add up how many carbs are in each ingredient in the entire recipe. Take the total carb content of the whole recipe and divide that amount by how many servings you plan to portion out.

That gives you the number of carbohydrate grams per serving.

Therefore, plain <u>Vanilla Custard Flan Cake</u> works out like this:

½ box cream cheese, softened but cool.................0 carbohydrate grams
2 eggs...0 carbohydrate grams
1/4 cup cornstarch..56 carbohydrate grams
OR whole-wheat flour, 1/4 cup............ ....OR. 23 carbohydrate grams
1 teaspoon real vanilla.......................................2 carbohydrate grams
¾ cup Karo ....337 carbohydrate grams
1 teaspoon non-aluminum baking powder............0 carbohydrate grams
<u>Total grams per this recipe...................................395 with cornstarch</u>

Divide 395 total grams by 6 servings = ~65 grams carbs per serving.

Divide 395 total grams by 8 servings = ~50 grams carbs per serving.

Divide 395 total grams by 12 servings = ~33 grams per serving.

This information is not already given for each recipe because sugar and carb quantities depend on your choice of ingredients, products and serving sizes.

(CAMPING)

PICNIC TABLE WORKOUT

1. **Find a sturdy, park-type picnic table.**
   Wipe off any animal poop, water, branches, etc.
   Put weights (cans of food, etc.) on table top for later.

2. **Stand at one end of the table**
   Slanted push-ups on the table ends
   Calf and Achilles tendon stretches
   Pull your bent leg up behind you and slowly stretch hamstrings

3. **Sit on bench. Face outwards**
   Feel your muscles relax as you reach further and further
   Head circles, side to side, chin out / in
   Leg lifts, bicycling, toe tapping
   Ankle mobility: feet up, down and all around
   - ❖ Bend forward—stretch down, sit up slowly.
   - ❖ Stand up. Sit down. Repeat
   - ❖ Raise arms up forward; sideways; repeat
   - ❖ Stretch to the left over your head, now to the right
   - ❖ Reach to the right behind you and then to the left
   - ❖ Reach over your head and down behind you with both arms.
   - ❖ *Weights: repeat the above exercises using hand weights*

4. **Walk around the table**
   Then sit, stretch it out to the left, ground and right.
   Reverse & repeat.
   You can do the same with hand weights.

5. **Walks/Hikes (with or without a furry friend)**
   Whatever distance and duration works for you.
   Wear good shoes; carry water, doggy scoop bags & tissues.

CONVERT U.S. MEASURES TO METRIC

(Rounding suggested below) is reasonable for these recipes—adjust if needed. This rule of thumb (heuristic) worked fine for us in Berlin, Germany.

If You Know This	Multiply It By	To Get
teaspoons	4.93 **(5)**	milliliters
Tablespoons	14.79 **(15)**	milliliters
fluid ounces	29.57 **(30)**	milliliters
cups	236.59 **(250)**	milliliters
cups	0.236 **(0.25)**	liters
pints	473.18 **(500)**	milliliters
pints	0.473 **(0.5)**	liters
quarts	946.36 **(1000)**	milliliters
quart	0.946 **(1)**	liter
gallons	3.785 **(4)**	liters
ounces	28.35 **(30)**	grams
pounds	0.454 **(0.5)**	kilograms
2 pounds	0.908 **(1)**	kilogram
inches	2.54 **(2.5)**	centimeters
Fahrenheit	subtract 32, multiply by 5 and divide by 9	Celsius (Centigrade)

CONVERT U.S. QUANTITIES

3 teaspoons per Tablespoon
16 Tablespoons per cup
48 teaspoons per cup
8 fluid ounces per cup
2 Tablespoons per ounce
1 ounce=1 standard "jigger" or "shot"
6 teaspoons per ounce

COUNTING CARBOHYDRATES

<u>Rule of Thumb Guidelines</u>: Carbohydrates (starches and sugars) raise blood sugar quickly, even whole grains. *Find more:* at www.carbcounter.org

Quantities below contain about 15 grams of "carbs" each.

STARCHES:
Bagel 1/4
Beans, dried, cooked 1/2 cup
Biscuit, 2-1/2"
Bread, white, wheat, rye, 1 slice
Cereal, cold 3/4 cup
Cereal, hot 1/2 cup
Chips, regular 9-13
Chips, tortilla 15-20
Cornbread 1-3/4" cube
Couscous 1/3 cup
Crackers, Round, 6
English muffin 1/2
Flour, any kind 1/8 cup
Graham crackers, 2" square
Granola 1/4 cup
Hamburger bun 1/2
Hot dog bun 1/2
Pancake or Waffle 4"
Pasta, cooked 1/3 cup
Pita pocket 6"
Pizza, thin crust 1 slice
Pretzels ¼ ounce
Rice, all types 1/3 cup
Roll, plain 1 small
Saltines 6
Split peas, cooked 1/2 cup
Squash: acorn, butternut 1/2 cup
Tortilla, all types 6"
Waffle or Pancake 4"

STARCHY VEGETABLES:
Corn on cob, 1/2 cob
Corn, cooked 1/2 cup
Corn, popped 3 cups
Hominy, canned 1/4 cup
Peas, cooked 1/2 cup
Plantain 1/3 cup
Potato 1 small, 1/4 large
Potato, boiled 1/2 cup or 1/2 med
Potato chips 1 oz.
Potato, French fried 1 cup
Yam/sweet potato 1/2 cup

DAIRY/MILK/YOGURT
Milk 1 cup (any fat level)
Yogurt, plain 1/2 - 2/3 cup

FRUIT (fructose sugar only)
Berries 1 cup
Canned 1/2 cup
Juice, all fruits 1/2 cup
Melon 1 cup
Raisins 2 Tablespoons
Raw fruit, large 1/2
Raw fruit, small, 1
Lemon juice: 1 oz.=3 grams carbs
      6 ounces 3/4 cup=15 gms carbs

SUGARS
Glucose syrup 3 teaspoons
Table sugar/fructose 4 teaspoons
Honey 3 teaspoons
www.carbcounter.org

CRAFTS
Made with food items

Easter Egg Sugar Molds
(can be eaten, but not recommended)

4 cups white sugar
2 egg whites

Mix well and press into several Pam-sprayed plastic egg molds, the kind that open from side to side, not top to bottom.
Carefully tip out onto a cookie sheet.

Bake 10 minutes at 200°F, then carefully scoop out inside (can re-use this sugar mixture) –

Flatten a bottom side while still soft. Cut peephole while still soft.

Let cool. Make a cute scene inside using plastic animals, etc. Then use pastry tubes to assemble with buttercream frosting. Can use frosting tubes.

Craft Dough to Bake
(NOT edible due to amount of salt)

2 cups white flour
1 cup salt
1 cup water, added gradually

Mix well. Knead 10 minutes or so. Can tint with food color. Make ornaments or crafts. Bake at 300°F until dry and hard. Paint, shellac, etc.

Play Dough to Stay Soft
(NOT edible due to amount of salt)

1 cup white flour
1/2 cup salt
1 cup water—if desired, tint water with food coloring (before cooking).
1 Tablespoons cooking oil
2 teaspoon cream of tartar

Mix in heavy saucepan, cook until mix forms a ball.
Store in plastic bag/or plastic container and keep in fridge. This will stay soft and workable a long time in an airtight container.

CRAFTS
Made with food items

Basic Papier-Maché
(paper muh**shey**)
(NOT recommended for eating)

Rip up a quantity of newspaper (don't use slick pages) into easily-handled pieces.

Put a cup or so of **white flour** into a shallow bowl or pie dish. Add water slowly and mix well until slightly runny

Dip newspaper pieces into wet flour until coated, and lay over chosen form, such as an inflated balloon suspended on a string from a hook or light fixture over a work area or table (work surface can be protected with plastic sheet, newspapers, etc.). Flatter or non-hollow forms should be held off the surface with pencils, dowels or sticks of some kind.

Keep adding layers of wet, flour-soaked newspaper until you decide it's thick enough. Allow to dry thoroughly. If using a balloon to make a hollow form, such as for a piñata, you can now pop the balloon with a pin and cut a 3-sided door, leaving 4th side attached as a hinge.

You can sand your form if desired to make it more smooth...decorate with paint, crepe paper, sparkles, whatever you desire.

To attach trim and decorations, Tacky Glue sets up much faster than regular school glue.

You can paint, varnish, shellac, or use other products as desired.

FRYING OILS AND FATS, SMOKE POINTS

Unrefined Canola Oil & Flaxseed Oil	225°F
Unrefined Safflower Oil & Sunflower Oil	225°F
Unrefined Corn & High-Oleic Sunflower Oil	320°F
Unrefined Olive Oil & Peanut Oil	320°F
Semi-Refined Safflower & Unrefined Soy Oil	320°F
Unrefined Walnut Oil	320°F
Shortening, Emulsified Vegetable	325°F
Hemp Seed Oil	330°F
Butter & Semi-refined Canola & Soy Oil	350°F
Unrefined Sesame Oil	350°F
Vegetable Shortening	360°F
Lard	370°F
Olive Oil	375°F
Macadamia Nut Oil	389°F
Canola l, Refined & Walnut Oil, Semi-Refined	400°F
Olive Oil, Extra Virgin*	406°F
Corn Oil & Sesame Oil	410°F
Cottonseed Oil & Grapeseed Oil	420°F
Coconut Oil (some up to)	425°F
Olive Oil, Virgin	435°F
Olive Oil & Rapeseed Oil	438°F
Peanut Oil & Sunflower Oil	440°F
Corn, Safflower, & Soy Oil, Refined	450°F
Peanut Oil, Refined	450°F
Sesame & Sunflower Oil, Semi-Refined	450°F
Olive Pomace Oil	460°F
Olive Oil, Extra Light	468°F
Grapeseed Oil	485°F
Soy Bean Oil	495°F
Safflower Oil	510°F
Avocado Oil, Refined	520°F

HEALTHIEST FOODS
Best From-the-Internet January 2016

1. Leafy vegetables
    Kale
    Spinach (gout alert, high purine)
    Broccoli
2. Nuts
    Peanuts, peanut butter, walnuts, almonds, etc.
    Cashews: higher in carbohydrates than most
3. Blueberries and other dark berries & cherries
4. Broad beans
    Navy, kidney, black, lima, etc.
5. Omega Three Fatty Acids
    Salmon
    Flax seed & flax seed meal or flax oil
    Oily fish (possible gout alert, some fish have high purine)
6. Poultry
7. Real olive oil
    Such as California Olive Ranch and others. See MoneyTalksNews
8. Red wine/dark grapes (wine—gout alert)
9. Tomatoes
    Including ketchup
    (Not in metal cans. Bottles or jars, OK)

PICNIC POSSIBILITIES

Some low-sugar suggestions

Devilled eggs, plain or spicy
Party meatballs, Mixed Meatballs
Fried chicken (without bones)
Dodo's cheesy bits
Nuts
Pickles
Ham & Asparagus Rollups
Cheese sticks & cubes
Fruit, whole, raw:
    Raw apples or oranges (sectioned), etc.
    Fruit Salad
Popcorn, popped & seasoned
Sandwiches:
    Flying fish sandwich
    Peanut butter and butter sandwich
    Meatloaf sandwich
    No-sugar lunchmeat sandwich
    Roast beef sandwich
    Chicken or turkey sandwiches
Vegetables
    Carrot or Celery sticks
    Broccoli or Cauliflower florets
    Cherry tomatoes
    Raw, bite-size vegetables, crudités
    Dip (ranch, bleu cheese, Salsaful, etc.)
    Olives
Grammy's surprise cake cubes, without drizzle
Drinks: water, milk, coffee, tea, Aztec cocoa

☠ POISONOUS TO DOGS ☠
This is not a complete list of all substances toxic to dogs!
If your pet has eaten any substances that may be poisonous, call:
ASPCA POISON CONTROL HOTLINE: 1-888-426-4435
NATIONAL PET POISON HELPLINE: 1-800-213-6680

- **Acetaminophen (Tylenol, Advil):** Gastric ulcers, kidney failure, death
- **Alcohol:** intoxication, coma, death
- **Avocado:** contains persin—vomiting, diarrhea
- **Bones, cooked:** stomach lacerations
- **Caffeine (tea, coffee, cocoa, chocolate):** toxic to heart & nervous system, vomiting, diarrhea
- **Chocolate (cocoa):** toxic to heart and nervous system, death
- **Cooked bones:** stomach lacerations
- **Currants (raisins & grapes, too):** kidney failure
- **Dairy (cow's milk):** too much: diarrhea, gastro-intestinal upset
- **Fat:** too much—pancreatitis, death
- **Fish:** many fish contain mercury. Multiple system problems, death.
- **Garlic:** blood cell damage—anemia
- **Grapes (currants & raisins):** kidney failure
- **Macadamia nuts:** nervous system & muscle damage
- **Marijuana:** moderate to severe toxicity to dogs (and cats, etc.)
- **Medications (Tylenol, Advil, other human prescription meds):** gastric ulcers, kidney failure, death
- **Milk** (dogs can be lactose-intolerant): too much: diarrhea, stomach upset
- **Mushrooms:** some varieties: shock & death—best to avoid all kinds
- **Onions (& garlic):** blood cell damage—anemia
- **Raisins (currants & grapes, too):** kidney failure
- **Salmon, raw:** often contains dangerous parasites.
- **Walnuts:** nervous system & muscle damage
- **Xylitol** (in gum, candy, toothpaste, etc.): liver failure, hypoglycemia, death

If your pet has ingested anything that may be poisonous, call:
ASPCA POISON CONTROL HOTLINE: 1-888-426-4435
NATIONAL PET POISON HELPLINE: 1-800-213-6680
☠ **This is not a complete list of all substances toxic to dogs!** ☠

PROPERLY BALANCED MEAL

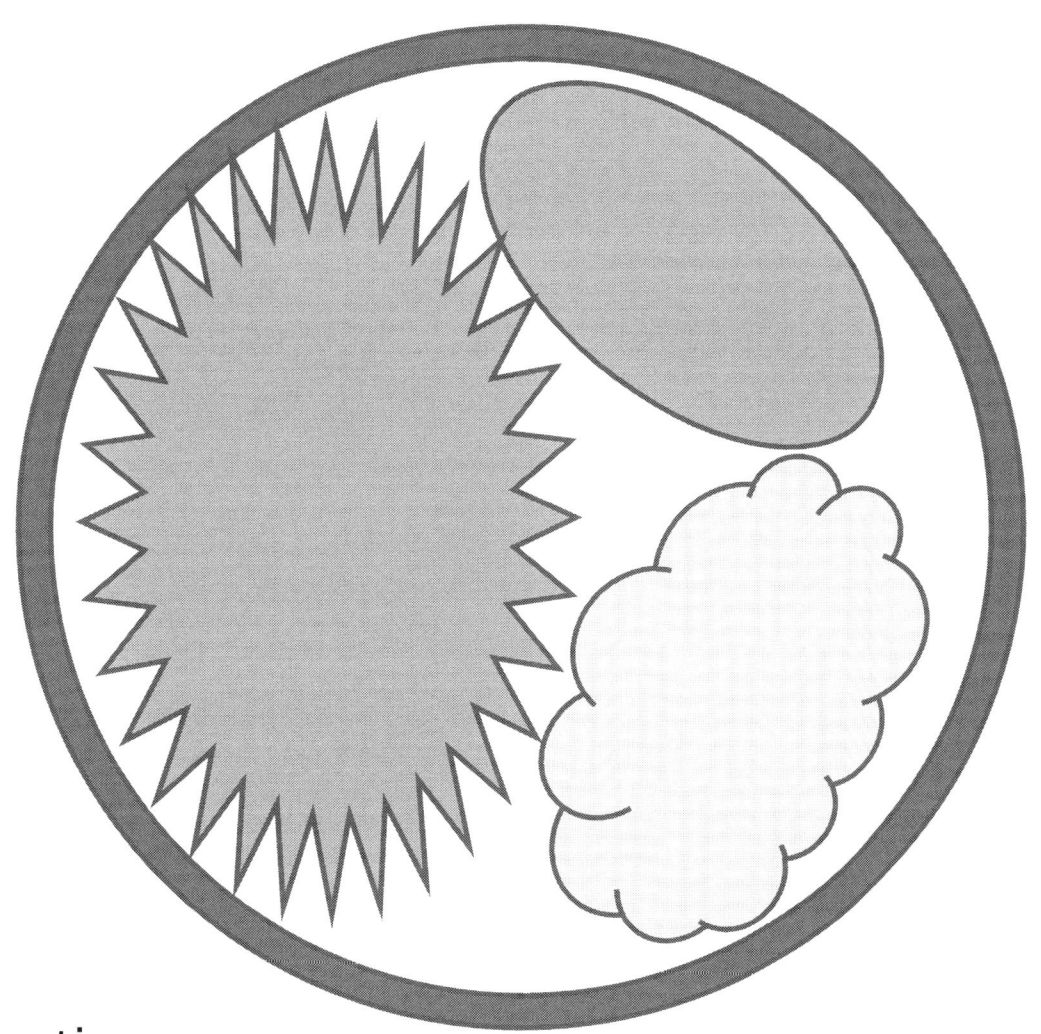

Suggestions:

1/2 plate= non-starchy vegetables, salad, non-sugared fruit
1/4 plate= starchy vegetables or grains including potatoes, rice, bread
1/4 plate= protein, including tofu, meat, fish, or poultry

VEGETARIAN: See Diet for a Small Planet or other vegetarian books for advice and recipes for a healthful, non-meat diet (eating complete proteins is very important).

TYPE II DIABETICS could reverse meat and vegetable quantities and may eliminate starchy/carbohydrate foods almost entirely. Talk with your doc.

SMALLER DISHES: if you eat from somewhat smaller plates, bowls, and drinkware, you'll almost automatically eat less and feel just about as full. Don't shrink your dishes too far. You can only be fooled visually just so much.

RECIPE VERSATILITY & ADAPTATION

    These recipes can be made in a variety of ways. For some we've indicated options, such as a number of flavor choices for EZ ice cream.
    Many ingredients are optional. Alter recipes to suit your own taste.
    Some recipes, however, require certain things to be worth making. If you leave the cream out of the ice cream, for example, it's no longer ice cream.
    Once we turned away from "sugar" recipes, the amount of fairly pricey Karo syrup required seemed high. But the cost made us far more aware of portion sizes, which is always vital—and often overlooked when baking with cheap white sugar.
    Your willingness to experiment with exact quantities and ingredients will help shape your satisfaction with eating **free-fructose free** and staying with it.

Adapting Recipes

1. Substitute 1-1/2 - 2 times as much Karo (or other glucose-only sugars) for table sugars, honey, etc...
   The Counting Carbohydrates chart shows that "sugar" contains 15 carb grams per 4 <u>teaspoons</u>, while glucose contains 15 carb grams per 3 teaspoons.
   Fructose-bearing sugars can be replaced by glucose sugars.
   It takes somewhat more glucose sugars to equal the same sweetness of fructose-bearing sugars. Whenever eating sugars or starches (carbohydrates), portion sizes really matter.

2. Add a bit more of the dry ingredients.

3. Cooking or baking times may need to be adjusted.

4. The dessert recipes here have already been altered. One, **Apple Crisp**, is shown both ways for an example of how to adapt a recipe.

REDUCING ADDED SUGARS & FRUCTOSE

Recipes are NOT low-calorie and don't produce or promote weight loss.

Most of these recipes follow guidelines from Dr. Robert Lustig's <u>FAT CHANCE</u> and <u>The Fat Chance Cookbook.</u> They have higher fiber, zero table sugar, and zero added or "free" fructose. They are more healthful alternatives to many recipes in <u>All Grammy's Best Recipes</u>.

Read labels. Check ingredient list and compare to the **69 Names of Sugar** Chart on page 107.

<u>**Karo Light**</u>, **Non-High-Fructose Corn Syrup** now says Non-HFCS on the front label. High Fructose Corn Syrup (HFCS) is composed of between 45%/55% and 25%/75% glucose to fructose ratio. Table sugars have a ratio of about a 50% glucose to 50% fructose, but glucose sugar is 100% glucose, with no fructose. Often Karo in the largest containers is high fructose corn syrup for candy makers and others whose recipes call for it specifically. Read labels!

Ketchup is problematic. You can find HFCS-free, but it will contain table sugar, which contains fructose (50%). Reduced-sugar ketchups contain artificial sweeteners, like sucralose, which should also be used with caution. Ketchup recipes so far have proved disappointing. Kicking a life-long ketchup relationship was almost as hard as kicking sugar itself.

Mayonnaise—the real kind has no added sugars. "Salad dressing" such as Miracle Whip, does contain added, fructose-containing sugars.

Any foods with added sugar--even glucose-only sweetened foods—are best eaten in limited quantities.

This book is not sponsored by Karo. ANY all-glucose sweetener will do,
As will any of the non-fructose sugars on the <u>69 Names of Sugar</u> list.

RELATIVE DAIRY FAT CONTENT

Milk, Half-and-Half Cream, Butter & Lard

Skim or Non-fat milk: 0.0 – 0.5% fat
1% or low-fat milk: about 1% fat
2% Milk: about 2% fat
Whole or Regular Milk: 3.25% fat
Half-and-Half: 10.5 – 18% fat
Light Cream: 18 – 30%% fat
Light Whipping Cream: 30% fat
Whipping Cream: 30 - 36% fat
Heavy Cream: 36 - 38% fat
Heavy Whipping Cream: 38 - 40% fat
Butter: 80% fat
Lard: 100% fat

Fat information & exact terms vary somewhat by source.

SIXTY-NINE NAMES OF SUGAR

(There are only 3 basic kinds of sugar: fructose, glucose, and lactose—<u>FAT CHANCE</u> by Dr. Lustig.)
(*with star = contains fructose, the slow toxin)
<u>(Bold, No star = glucose or lactose)</u>

Agave nectar*
Barbados sugar*
Barley malt=glucose
Beet sugar*
Blackstrap molasses*
Brown rice syrup*
Brown sugar*
Buttered syrup*
Cane juice crystals*
Cane sugar* (50/50)
Caramel*
Carob syrup*
Castor sugar*
Confectioners' sugar*
Corn sugar* (read labels!)
Corn syrup, Light=glucose
Corn syrup solids=glucose
Crystalline fructose*
Date sugar*
Demerara sugar*
Desiccated cane syrup*
Dextran
Dextrin=glucose
Dextrose=glucose
Diastatic malt=glucose
Diatase=glucose
Ethyl maltol=glucose
Evaporated cane juice*
Florida crystals*
Fructose* (100% fructose)
Fruit juice* (100% fructose)
Fruit juice concentrate* (fructose)
Galactose=milk sugar=lactose
Glucose
Glucose solids

Glucose syrup
Golden sugar*
Golden syrup*
Grape sugar*
High-fructose corn syrup*
HFCS* (45% glucose/55% fructose)
High Maltose Corn Syrup=glucose
HMCS (High Maltose Corn Syrup)
Honey*
Icing sugar*
Invert sugar*
Lactose=milk sugar
Levulose*
Malt syrup=glucose
Maltodextrin=glucose/dextrin
Maltose=glucose
Maple syrup*
Molasses*
Muscovado sugar*
Organic raw sugar*
Panocha*
Powdered Sugar*
Raw sugar*
Refiner's syrup*
Refinery syrup*
Rice syrup=glucose
Sorghum syrup*
Sucrose* (50% glucose, 50% fructose)
Sugar* (50/50)
Table sugar* (50/50)
Tomato juice* (100% fructose)
Treacle*
Turbinado sugar*
Yellow sugar*
<u>Fructose is great plant fertilizer!</u>

Suggested Reading

Dr. Robert Lustig: *FAT CHANCE*
Highly Recommended

Cindy Gershen and Robert Lustig*:*
The FAT Chance Cookbook

William Dufty: *Sugar Blues*

David Gillespie*: Sweet Poison*

John Yudkin: *Pure, White, and Deadly*

http://carb-counter.org/
Good counts online of
carbohydrates, fiber, & more

Summarized Fast Food Carbohydrate Guidelines

McDonald's & *Taco Time* Nutrition Data Sheets 2016

BEVERAGES	CARBOHYDRATE GRAMS
Milk	12
Small Diet Coke / Large Dr. Pepper	*0 / 120*
BREAKFASTS	**CARBOHYDRATE GRAMS**
Apple/Cinnamon/Walnut Oatmeal	45
Bagels / Biscuits / English Muffins	55 / 40 / 30
Big Breakfast with English Muffin	41
Big Breakfast w/Pancakes	111
Burritos / McMuffins / Hash Browns	26 / 30 / 15
Muffins with fruit baked in	60-65
Pancakes (3) / Syrup (1)	60 / 45
Portuguese sausage eggs & rice	37
FISH	**CARBOHYDRATE GRAMS**
Filet O' Fish: Bay / Regular / Double	41 / 39 / 49
Fish Baja (2) / Fish Soft Taco	*35 / 77*
SALADS	**CARBOHYDRATE GRAMS**
Bacon Ranch Salad w/chicken	10 grilled 24 crispy
Dressing: S.W. / Ranch / Italian	11
Dressing: Balsamic Vinaigrette	5
Dressing: French / Thousand Island	22
Dressing: Guacamole / Corn Salsa	*3 / 10*
Whole Black Beans / Sour Cream	*32 / 4*
Side Salad / Croutons	4 / 10
Southwest Salad	28 grilled / 43 crispy
Chicken Caesar Salad with dressing	*15*
Chicken Taco Salad no dressing	*22*
Chicken Tostado Salad no dressing	*52*
Cilantro Lime Chicken Salad	*28*
SIDES	**CARBOHYDRATE GRAMS**
Apple Slices / Pineapple	4 / 15
French Fries / Ketchup	15 / 30 / 45 / 70 / 2 each pkt.

Mexi-Fries Small/Medium/Large	*21 / 43 / 64*
Chips & Salsa	*64*
Popcorn	25 small / 55 large
DESSERTS	**CARBOHYDRATE GRAMS**
Yogurt / GoGurt	24 / 30 w. granola / 9 topping
Pies / Ice Cream per scoop	33 / 30
Chocolate Chip / Oatmeal Cookie	22 / 22
Coffee Cake / Carmel Apple Parfait	27 / 33
Crustos / Churro Bites	*30 / 45*
CHICKEN	**CARBOHYDRATE GRAMS**
Chicken McNuggets	6/18 10/30 20/59 40/118
Chicken Selects, Southern Style (3)	20
Chicken Wraps, Snack / Regular	30 / 60
McChicken / Deluxe / Crispy	40 / 48 / 59
Sauce: Honey Mustard	6
Sauce: Ranch / BBQ / Sweet & Sour	12
White Chicken Chili Cup / Bowl	*24/ 72*
SANDWICHES, WRAPS, TACOS	**CARBOHYDRATE GRAMS**
Bacon Cheese / Bacon Double	35
Big Mack / Quarter Pounder BLT	47
Cheeseburger, Double/ Triple	33 / 36
Hamburger / Double / Homestyle	32 / 35 / 38
McRib / Tender Pork & Gravy	45 / 42
Quarter Pounder / Double	39 / 49
Quarter Pounder Bacon Club	52
Southern Style chicken Sandwich	43
Crisp Burrito: Bean / Beef / Chicken	*41 / 27 / 23 /*
Veggie Classic Burrito	*89*
Beef classic Burrito	*92*
Soft Habanero Chicken Burrito	*84*
Crisp Taco: Bean / Beef / Chicken	*20 / 15 / 10*
Soft Taco: Veggie / Beef Natural	*71 / 61*
Soft Taco:PintoBean/ChickenCaesar	*79 / 59*

Values from McDonald's & *Taco Time* 2016 Nutrition Charts

INDEX

Appetizers & Snacks..11
- Buttermilk Cheese Dip—14
- Chips—12
- Creamy/Dilly Dip—13
- Crudités—14
- DIY Microwave Popcorn—15
- Dodo's Cheesy Bits—12
- Ham & Asparagus Rollups—11
- Kimmy's Hamburger Dip—13
- Pappa's Antique Popcorn--15
- Salsaful Chip & Veg Dip—12
- Spicy Sweet Party Meatballs—11

Beverages..16
- Coffee & Tea—16
- Dodo's Antique Eggnog—Updated—16
- Hot Cocoa, Aztec & Swiss—16
- Juice & Carbonation—17
- Milk—17
- Water--17

Bird Food..18
- Hummingbird Nectar—18
- Suet—18

Breads..19
- A Few Store-Bought Whole Grain Breads—24
- Bannock Bread—23
- Cornbread—19
- Dodo's Celery & Onion Holiday Stuffing—22
- Flat Bread—21
- Holiday Bread Bowls—19
- Whole Grain Bounce—20

Camping..25
- Double-Baked Potato Boat--26
- Hurry-Up Casserole—26
- New Breed of Dog—25

Camping, Continued
    Scrapple—27

Casseroles 28
    Bubble & Squeak—28
    Grandma's German Chili—29
    Harvest Casserole—28
    Southwest Casserole—30

Dog Food & Treats 31
    Basic Dog Food—32
    Doggy Cookies—33
    Eggshell Powder—32
    Hi-Pro Kibble Cookies—35
    Most Popular Human Foods 4 Dogs—31
    Pumpkin Treats—34
    Store-Bought Dog Food Feeding Guide—32
    Sweet Yam Chews—34

Dog Food: Puppy Formula & Feeding 36
    Puppy Feeding Schedule—36
    Supplemental & Replacement—36

Eggs, Pancakes, & Breakfast 37
    Creamy Devilled Eggs—37
    Dodo's Eggy Pancakes—39
    Microwave Omelet—39
    Pancake Toppings—40
    Pappa's Perfect Omelet—38
    Quiche Eileen—38
    Spicy Devilled Eggs—37
    Traditional Steel-cut Oats—41
    Whole Grain Pancakes—40

Fish 42
    Ahi Tuna Steaks—42
    Battered Fish Fillets—43
    Salmon: Baked—43, Broiled—42
    Unfishy Fried Fish—42

Fruit 44
    Fried Apples—44

Marinades..**45**
    Cooked Marinade—45
    Refrigerator Marinade—45

Meat...**46**
    Meat-Stuffed Acorn Squash—51
    Microwaved Bacon—47
    Microwaved Ground Meat—51
    Mixed Meat Patties—49
    Modern Meatloaf—47
    New Breed of Dog—50
    Pork Loin Surprise—48
    Sausage Suggestion—48
    Schnitzel—46
    Simple Enchiladas—46
    Swedish Meatballs—50

Nutritional Information
    About Sweeteners—9
    Calculate Carb Grams per Serving—93
    (Camping) Picnic Table Workout—94
    Convert U.S. Measures to Metric & Convert Quantities—95
    Counting Carbohydrates—96
    Crafts—97
    Frying Oils & Fats, Smoke Points—99
    Healthiest Foods 2016—100
    Picnic Possibilities—101
    Poisonous to Dogs—102
    Properly Balanced Meal—103
    Recipe Versatility & Adaptation—104
    Reducing Added Sugars & Fructose—105
    Relative Dairy Fat Contents—106
    Sixty-nine Names of Sugar—107
    Suggested Reading—108
    Summarized Fast Food Carbohydrate Guidelines—109
    Vegetables & Insulin—92
    Index—111

Pasta..**52**
    Grammy's Best Lasagna—52
    Green Cheese Rotini—53
    The Family Spaghetti—54

Polenta..**55**
    Cheesy Polenta—55
    What is Polenta?—55

Potatoes..**56**
    Cheddar & Bacon Potato Salad—57
    Dodo's Antique Potato Salad—56
    Dodo's Potato Pancakes—58
    Latkes—56
    Microwaved Bakers—58
    Stuffed Potatoes—58
    Twice-Baked Potatoes—57

Poultry..**59**
    Chicken Piccata—60
    Chicken Quesadillas—61
    Dodo's Antique 2-Step Chicken—62
    Fried Chicken—61
    Grandpa Gene's Chicken Cacciatore—59
    Hawaiian Chicken Salad Mountain—62
    Microwaved Chicken—59

Rice...**63**
    Plain Rice Cooking Chart—63
    Chop Suey—64
    Spanish Rice--63

Salads & Dressings...**65**
    Andrea's Spinach Mandarin Salad, Party-Size—69
    Buttermilk Cheese Dressing—66
    Creamy Dressing—66
    Creamy Ranch Dressing—65
    Crunchy Cabbage Salad—67
    Grammy's Caesar Salad—68
    Greek Salad—67

Salads & Dressings, Continued
- Lovely Pea Salad--69
- Pappa's Basic Leafy Salad—68
- Pasta Salad Italiano—67
- Salsaful Dressing—66
- Vinaigrette/Italian Dressing—65

Sandwiches...70
- Basic Croque Madam—71
- Basic Croque Monsieur—71
- Basic PB&J—72
- Basic Welsh Rabbit—72
- Cold Flying Fish Sandwich—70
- Hot Flying Fish Melt—70
- Hot French Dip==72

Slow Cooker...73
- Bar-B-Que—73
- Roast & Stew—73
- Stroganoff—74
- Swiss Steak--74

Soups...75
- Alma's Pozole—76
- Artesian Tomato Soup—76
- Cheryl's Yin Yang Soup—79
- Clam Chowder—77
- Fresh Broccoli Soup—78
- Fresh Carrot Soup—78
- Pappa Paul's Green Veg Soup—75
- Pappa Paul's Red Veg Soup—75

Sweets (Desserts, Treats, & Snacks)..80
- Autumn Ice Cream—85
- Cake Toppings—82
- Cheesecake, Three Ways—87
    - Both Worlds—87
    - Cake Style—87
    - Custard Style—87

Sweets: Desserts, Treats, & Snacks, Continued
- Chocolate Flannel Moose—82
- EZ Homemade Ice Cream—86
- Flavors 4 Ice Cream or Toppings—86
- Fresh Heavenly Hash—84
- Fresh Strawberries Luella—83
- Grammy's 1967-2017 Apple Crisp—83
- Holiday Pumpkin Cheesecake Pie—85
- Mousse Cake—80
- Oatseed Cake—81
- Plain Cake—80
- Pumpkin Pie Spice—895
- Relative Cost 4 Ice Cream—086
- Very Berry Whip—84

Vegetables..88
- Cheese-Stuffed Mushrooms—88
- Cheesy Beans—89
- Cooking Chart (vegetables cooked many ways)—90 - 91
- Easy-Peasy Coleslaw—88
- Multi-Bean Salad (3-Bean Salad)—89
- Roasted Brussels Sprouts—88
- *Vegetables & Insulin—92*

About the authors:

Kathleen Krauss Zucati
was born in Hillsboro, Oregon
back when pterodactyls darkened the skies.
Her father was a cook in the US National Guard.
She grew up in the Pacific Northwest, was educated
at the University of Puget Sound, and is a member of OATHS.
She lives with her first husband, Paul,
and two entitled pug girls.
She has low vision.
She is Grammy.

Paul Edward Zucati,
was born in Chehalis, Washington, at age zero.
His father was a professional cook, both US Navy and civilian,
Paul has been cooking since he was six years old, standing on a box.
In our kitchen, he's the chief cook and bottle washer.
He lives with his first wife, Kathleen,
and two entitled pug girls.
He is Pappa.

LARGE PRINT
for easier reading

Made in the USA
San Bernardino, CA
12 May 2017